Messengers of Sex

Since the early twentieth century, hormones have commonly been understood as 'messengers of sex'. They are seen as essential to the development and functioning of healthy reproductive male and female bodies; millions take them as medications in the treatment of fertility, infertility and aging. However, in contemporary society, hormones are both disturbed and disturbing; invading our environments and bodies through plastics, food and water, environmental oestrogens and other chemicals, threatening irreversible, inter-generational bodily change. Using a wide range of sources, from physiology textbooks to popular parenting books and pharmaceutical advertisements, Celia Roberts analyses the multiple ways in which sex hormones have come to matter to us today. Bringing feminist theories of the body into dialogue with science and technology studies, she develops tools to address one of the most important questions facing feminism today: how is biological sex conceivable?

CELIA ROBERTS is a Lecturer in the Department of Sociology at Lancaster University. She is the co-author of *Born and Made: An Ethnography of Preimplantation Genetic Diagnosis* (with Sarah Franklin, 2006).

Cambridge Studies in Society and the Life Sciences

Series Editors
Nikolas Rose, *London School of Economics*
Paul Rabinow, *University of California at Berkeley*

This interdisciplinary series focuses on the social shaping, social meaning and social implications of recent developments in the life sciences, biomedicine and biotechnology. It places original research and innovative theoretical work within a global, multi-cultural context.

Messengers of Sex

Hormones, biomedicine and feminism

CELIA ROBERTS
Lancaster University

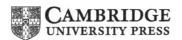

CAMBRIDGE
UNIVERSITY PRESS

CAMBRIDGE
UNIVERSITY PRESS

University Printing House, Cambridge CB2 8BS, United Kingdom

Cambridge University Press is part of the University of Cambridge.

It furthers the University's mission by disseminating knowledge in the pursuit of education, learning and research at the highest international levels of excellence.

www.cambridge.org
Information on this title: www.cambridge.org/9780521681971

First published 2007

A catalogue record for this publication is available from the British Library

ISBN 978-0-521-68197-1 Paperback

Contents

Figures

A message to readers

Like mine, your worlds probably teem with messages: emails, text messages, answer-phone messages, targeted advertising. Arriving home, at work, off the plane, onto the train, we check our messages. Who has been in contact with us? What did they have to say? What do they want us to do?

These messages are both a boon and a burden. I can barely imagine academic or personal life without email, but often approach my inbox with trepidation, especially after avoiding it for several days. These forms of messaging carve novel channels of communication and make possible new ways of articulating love, hostility, demand and care. Messaging, we have all learnt in deeply embodied ways (the thud of your heart as you double-click to open an email; the delight on someone's face as they read a text message; the involuntary smile as you hear a recorded familiar voice), is neither bland nor purely technical. Messages do not just convey information; they implicate, stir up feeling, make new worlds and responsibilities, create personal and political dilemmas. In short, messages are actions and stimulate further actions.

In the midst of this early twenty-first-century proliferation of messages comes the demise of historically significant cultural forms of *messengers*. On 3 February 2006, for example, Western Union terminated its telegram services. Announced on the internet, this closure of a 150-year-old service made few waves. We no longer need human messengers and slips of paper to make contact; our machines perform these services, albeit with huge amounts of labour and vast investments of time and money to produce and maintain the related technologies. The messaging we are used to now appears to work without embodied messengers: messages move 'instantly' between the sender and the receiver. The technologies underlying contemporary messages are of course still material, but messengers today are distributed, made up of hard-to-grasp entities like software and silicon chips. The entities and networks that carry our messages are massively complex sets of relations between machines, humans, objects and codes. In contemporary forms of communication, then, messages are not entities carried from one place to another by an independent messenger. Messages flow through a complex network of relations and are literally constituted by these relations.

In biological terms too, we inhabit worlds brimming with messages. Most significant culturally are genes and chromosomes, which are often described as containing 'instructions' or 'codes' that are executed by cells. In pervasive popular discourses of genetic determinism, genes are described as carrying information through generations, instructing bodies to developmentally unfold physical and psychological characteristics, propensities for specific diseases and particular skills and attributes. In the case of sex, this role has been described scientifically as relatively simple: each human has two sex chromosomes coding for maleness or femaleness, a coding that produces gonadal differences *in utero* and initiates a cascade of sexual differences throughout foetal development and postnatal life. This representation is undermined by the fact that genes and chromosomes cannot work on their own; genetic 'instructions' must be 'carried out' by other biological entities such as neurons, hormones and proteins within complex biological and ecological systems. Increasingly, as science-studies theorist Joan Fujimura describes, scientists find that genes interact with other genes, 'with various proteins, developmental pathways, cell signalling pathways, and many other parts of cellular, organismal, and environmental parts and processes that are fast becoming the territory of a new field called "systems biology"' (Fujimura 2006: 28). Even in the supposedly relatively simple example of sex determination, then, technoscientific understandings of the messaging work of genes is 'steadily increasing in complexity' (Fujimura 2006: 28).

Alongside genes, hormones constitute one of the three most significant biological messaging systems for plants, animals and humans (the neurological system is the third one). Whilst a significant body of social scientific and cultural analysis of the messaging actions of genes has developed, there has been very little on hormones (or indeed neurons). This book, then, makes a contribution to social scientific and cultural analysis of contemporary biological actors by focusing on these less popular biological actors. In particular, it reworks the early twentieth-century idea of hormones as 'messengers of sex' to theorise the role of biology in the production of sexed bodies.

Messengers of Sex describes the historical development and contemporary state of technoscientific and biomedical understandings of hormonal action. In mainstream understandings, developed from the late nineteenth century onwards, hormones are understood to carry messages within sealed, homeostatic systems: systems that maintain a natural health or 'balance' in the body. Working with telegram-era models of messaging, early to mid-twentieth-century endocrinology understood the messenger as a non-implicated entity that carries a stable message from one preexisting and active entity to a responsive other. This conventional model describes sex hormones (oestrogen, progesterone and testosterone) as taking the message of 'sex' from the genes (which programme a predetermined sex) to the body (which changes according to the content of the message, thus producing bodily sexual difference). This model is represented in twentieth-century endocrinology textbooks and other technoscientific and popular literature in flow diagrams and line drawings of human bodies. Arrows represent the messaging of hormones moving in circular loops between the gonads (which are genetically programmed to produce sex hormones), the brain (where other hormones are produced) and other relevant parts of the body (to stimulate breast and body-hair growth during puberty, for example). These depictions borrow from mid-twentieth-century models of cybernetic signalling: hormonal circuits are figured as negative feedback loops in which the messages ('information') conveyed by hormones as 'inputs' change the activities or 'outputs' of the cells and organs at their destination.

In the early twenty-first century, this technoscientific model of hormonal action – like its information and communication technology counterparts – is undergoing serious stress-related change, caused by a kind of 'information overload'. This change provides an opportunity to reconsider conventional figurations of hormones as messengers of sex. In a review article, environmental toxicologist John McLachlan (2001) describes how early twentieth-century definitions of oestrogens are breaking down in the contemporary biosciences. In the first three decades of the twentieth century, 'oestrogen' came to refer to a chemical message that produces a period of heat (estrus) in a female animal or human. As the material practices of endocrinological research developed – from injecting chemicals into mice's vaginas or testing the weight of the uteruses of castrated mice, to microbiochemical analyses of how hormones move through the body and bind with specific receptor sites on the cell walls of target organs – this definition changed. Oestrogens came to be defined as 'chemicals capable of stimulating an increased number of cells from

oestrogen target organs grown in tissue culture; [or] chemicals that form
ligands [bonds] for the ER [oestrogen receptor] and displace radiolabeled
estradiol from its binding' (McLachlan 2001: 328). Even more recently, as
this work joined up with genetic research, hormones came to be understood as 'chemicals that regulate the expression of oestrogen target genes;
and, chemicals that transactivate ER-driven reporter genes in cells in
culture' (McLachlan 2001: 328).

These functional definitions of oestrogens, derived from specific technoscientific practices, today cause problems for scientists because increasing numbers of chemicals can be said to do *some* of these things, but not
others. McLachlan articulates these controversies: 'If a chemical binds the
ER with a high affinity and specificity, is it an oestrogen? Or must it also
activate ER-regulated genes? Must it lead to a functional response?'
(McLachlan 2001: 328). Such questions make some scientists want to
return to earlier certainties, to insist that 'oestrogens' must always stimulate the tissues of the female genital tract. Others are more open to the
suggestion that it is no longer clear what an oestrogen is. Semour
Lieberman (1996 cited in McLachlan 2001), for example, argues that one
of the bestknown naturally occurring substances in this field – estriol –
may *not* 'really' be an oestrogen, despite being called such for sixty years,
because it does not produce estrus. McLachlan describes this dilemma with
some glee. Lieberman, he writes, 'raises the deliciously provocative possibility that estriol, the oestrogen of pregnancy in humans, may actually
have a different role than one might surmise from its classification as
oestrogen' (McLachlan 2001: 328). Lieberman thus raises a significant,
disturbing question: 'When is an oestrogen an oestrogen, and when is it
not?'(Lieberman, in McLachlan 2001: 328).

McLachlan's interest in these definitional difficulties is fuelled by work
on endocrine-disrupting chemicals (or environmental oestrogens) and
their actions in plants, invertebrates, animals and humans. McLachlan's
and others' research on these chemicals challenges traditional definitions
of hormones and troubles modern understandings of the boundaries and
characteristics of the hormonally sexed body. As in the case of email and
text messaging, the volume of (hormonal) messages has recently massively
increased, causing confusion both about what a message is and how to
distinguish between a message and a messenger. McLachlan describes our
contemporary world as one of 'environmental signalling', in which chemicals of many sorts send messages to plants, insects, animals and humans,
encouraging genetic and cellular change of both profound (irreversible or
organisational) and acute (reversible or activational) kinds. Sex hormones,

McLachlan (2001: 319) argues, should now be understood as part of 'ecosystem-wide communication networks' that link numerous species, contributing to diverse forms of health and illness. This view is a long way from the sealed, homeostatic messaging systems of twentieth-century endocrinological thought described earlier.

In this book I elaborate this twenty-first-century uncertainty, making an argument for *reconfiguring* technoscientific understandings of sex hormones as messengers. In contrast to conventional biological models that suggest that hormones message something definite and known ('sex') between two already existing entities, I argue that the act of messaging constitutes both the sender and the receiver of the message and that messaging can be understood as a relationship or communication between the active entities thus constituted. The content of the message – 'sex' – is also not predetermined in this model.

This argument is made through a detailed investigation of the inter-relationship between arenas commonly described as 'the social' and 'the biological'. Critically considering key examples of hormones' messaging (how messaging happens in physiology textbooks, in animal and human bodies, in biomedicine and in popular culture), this book demonstrates how hormones actively participate in the enactment of particular versions of the biological (or nature) and the social (or culture) and of sex. I am convinced that because such enactments are historically specific materiali-sations (to use Judith Butler's term) or articulations (to use Donna Haraway's term), they could potentially be done in other ways, leading to other forms of biology/nature and the social/culture and, indeed, sex itself. This is the political aspect of this project: to investigate what is limiting about existing hormonal messaging and consider how to open space for variation or change.

This consideration of sex hormones is intrinsically linked with feminist politics. In the Introduction, I situate this book's argument about hormones in feminist debates about the biological or material body. Sex hormones have a complex history within feminism and have often been understood as negative constraints on women's endeavours. Engaging seriously with biological thinking in an attempt to challenge this negativ-ity, this book goes somewhat out on a limb in terms of feminism, which – a significant but small tradition of feminist science studies notwithstanding – has traditionally been wary of biological discourses of sex. Today, how-ever, this limb is not a particularly lonely spot; in an era dubbed 'The Century of Biology', feminist theorists (and many others) are increasingly turning their attention to such issues. Along with theorists such as Donna Haraway, Elizabeth Grosz and Rosi Braidotti – but in notably different ways – this book argues that feminism needs to theorise biological actors like hormones and to take seriously the multiple discourses that describe their actions in bodies. These actions articulate highly significant relationships between human and non-human actors – relationships that constitute contemporary forms of sexual difference and life itself. Like the messengers constituting our contemporary communication technologies, hormones establish complex and distributed embodied relations in ways barely perceptible to most of us that are both profoundly important and historically specific (and therefore contestable). This book tells critically engaged stories about hormones as messengers of sex in order to bring these actions to the surface and to articulate their relevance to feminist politics.

Acknowledgements

This book reflects two major periods of my academic and personal life: firstly, my doctoral research at the Department of Women's Studies at the University of Sydney and secondly, my time as a post-doctoral researcher and lecturer in the Department of Sociology at Lancaster University. At Sydney I had the great fortune to work with two inspiring intellectuals: historian Barbara Caine and philosopher Moira Gatens. It's been a long time since they supervised the earliest versions of this research, but their influence on this book and my work is still palpable. The interdisciplinary Department of Women's Studies fostered my interest in feminist theory and politics and gave me the opportunity to develop lasting friendships with wonderful feminist scholars: kylie valentine, Catherine Waldby, Mary Spongberg, Linnell Secomb, Kerry Sanders, Denise Russell, Noni Rummery and Suzanne Fraser amongst numerous others.

Moving to Lancaster reinvigorated my original training as a social scientist and developed my passion for the unusual combination of women's studies and science studies. Since 2001, I have enjoyed both the newness of 'being in Sociology' and engaging with the Institute for Women's Studies and the Centre for Science Studies. Many people made this a mind-expanding experience for me: Imogen Tyler, Lucy Suchman, Jackie Stacey, Vicky Singleton, Katrina Roen, Michal Nahman, Maggie Mort, Maureen McNeil, Gail Lewis, John Law, Hilary Hinds, Hilary Graham, Sarah Franklin, Anne-Marie Fortier, Anne Cronin, Cathy Clay, Claudia Casteñada and Sara Ahmed to name some key people. Lancaster has also provided the most extraordinary stream of visiting academics whose work has been inspiring: Rosi Braidotti, Barbara Duden, Donna Haraway, Amade M'charek, Ingunn Moser, Annemarie Mol and Anneke Smelik, amongst many others. My Ph.D., M.A. and undergraduate students have also taught me a lot about researching, writing and communicating. I hope some of them find things of interest in this book.

Numerous people helped me more specifically with this book project. Catherine Waldby was encouraging from the outset and assisted me in developing the proposal. Hilary Hinds nobly read the whole manuscript at a point of indirection and helped me see it afresh. Karen Throsby, Suzanne Fraser, Will Medd, Anne Cronin and kylie valentine generously gave detailed comments on chapters and Michal Nahman was always prepared to talk through the latest dilemma. Jackie Stacey kept me on track in difficult times and gave speedy and incisive feedback from afar. Adrian Mackenzie critically engaged with all the bits that had to be said out loud, as well as reading numerous chapter drafts. In the Sociology Department, Claire O'Donnell provided me with endlessly cheerful and practical administrative advice and assistance, whilst at Cambridge University Press, the anonymous reviewer and series editors Nikolas Rose and Paul Rabinow were encouraging and helpful, as were editors John Haslam and Carrie Cheek. Finally, finishing the manuscript in 2006 was made possible by a Research Leave Award granted by the Arts and Humanities Research Council, whose funding scheme for projects nearing completion is a godsend.

Alongside my academic friends are the other people who make thinking and working possible for me. In this regard, my heartfelt thanks to Hilary, Hugh and Tom Roberts and the rest of the Roberts family, Moya Mackenzie and the other Mackenzies, Ruth and Rex Burgess, David McMaster and Tim Kobin, Alison Ross and Amir Ahmadi, Mark Westcombe, Sabrina Mazzoni and Alison Mazoudier and all my 'old' school friends. Adrian Mackenzie mixes up my academic and 'other' worlds on a daily basis and will probably be the most pleased that this book is finally finished. After all, he was there when it started as a fledgling proposal.

Portions of this book are expanded and reworked versions of the following previously published articles: 'Biological Behavior? Hormones, Psychology and Sex', in *The Science and Politics of the Search for Sex Differences: A special issue of the NWSA journal*, 12(3) (2000): 1–20 reproduced by permission of Indiana University Press; '"A Matter of Embodied Fact": Sex Hormones and the History of Bodies', *Feminist Theory* 3(1) (2002): 7–26 and 'Drowning in a Sea of Estrogens: Sex Hormones, Sexual Reproduction and Sex', *Sexualities* 6(2) (2003): 195–213, reproduced by permission of Sage Publications Ltd. and '"Successful Aging" with Hormone Replacement Therapy: It may be sexist, but what if it works?' *Science as Culture* 11(1) (2002): 39–59. My thanks to the publishers for granting me permission to use this material.

Introduction: feminism, bodies and biological sex

In 1949 Simone de Beauvoir passionately described women's enslavement to what she called the 'outside forces' of their reproductive biologies. 'Woman is of all mammalian females', she wrote,

> at once the one who is most profoundly alienated (her individuality the prey of outside forces), and the one who most violently resists this alienation; in no other is enslavement of the organism to reproduction more imperious or more unwillingly accepted. Crises of puberty and the menopause, monthly 'curse', long and often difficult pregnancy, painful and sometimes dangerous childbirth, illnesses, unexpected symptoms and complications – these are characteristics of the human female.
>
> *(de Beauvoir 1988: 64)*

These crises are fundamentally linked to endocrine systems; for de Beauvoir, puberty, ovulation, menstruation, pregnancy, childbirth and menopause all demonstrate the ways in which 'the species' takes hold of women's bodies through the actions of sex hormones. Women's lives are a profound struggle against this 'imperious' process. 'Not without resistance', she argues, 'does the body of woman permit the species to take over; and this struggle is weakening and dangerous' (de Beauvoir 1988: 59). Unlike men (whose endocrine systems do not create significant crises), a woman must strive to maintain a hold on her individuality and resist her 'enslavement' to the demands of biological reproduction, which are, physiologically at least, of no benefit to her (de Beauvoir 1988: 62–4). 'Woman, like man', de Beauvoir argues with reference to the work of phenomenologist Maurice Merleau-Ponty, '*is* her body; but her body is something other than herself' (de Beauvoir 1988: 61, emphasis in original). To become herself, then, a woman must resist the inherent nature of her (hormonal) body, which is to sublimate her, like other mammals, to the reproduction of the species. Although her descriptions of this struggle are graphic, with the words

1

'enslavement' and 'imperious' figuring a desire for revolt against biological forces, de Beauvoir is adamant that hormones do not, as science writer Gail Vines (1993) puts it, 'rule our lives'. After stating that 'the biological facts ... are one of the keys to the understanding of woman', she continues 'I deny that they establish for her a fixed and inevitable destiny' (de Beauvoir 1988: 65). For de Beauvoir, women's subordinate role cannot be explained by biology, and indeed, as she famously contends much later in *The Second Sex*, 'One is not born, but rather becomes, a woman' (de Beauvoir 1988: 295).

This seeming contradiction in de Beauvoir's position – becoming a woman is a social/cultural process but women continually struggle against the powerful forces of biology – epitomises a continuing dilemma within feminist theory. To what extent are women's socially subordinate positions influenced by their biologies? And what are the possibilities for change or 'struggle' against biological 'forces'? At the heart of this dilemma lie shifting meanings of 'biology' and recurrent slippages between biology as a science and biology as body or material flesh. Holding these two versions of biology apart is notoriously difficult for both scientists and social theorists. De Beauvoir, for example, despite describing the scientific knowledge of her time as 'fact', points out that 'all physiologists and biologists ... ascribe meaning to vital phenomena' and often make 'foolhardy' deductions from biological data about animals in explaining human society (de Beauvoir 1988: 41, 45). Since the 1970s, feminist critics of science and medicine such as Ruth Hubbard, Linda Birke and Evelyn Fox Keller, have shown that the scientific discipline of biology is demonstrably cultural and political, its assertions value-laden and reductive. But the question of how this relates to biological bodies, to biology as material flesh, remains contested. If contemporary feminists want to resist women's 'enslavement' (to use de Beauvoir's word) to their biologies, we need, arguably, to do more than analyse the discipline of biology. De Beauvoir's assertion that there is something in the very materiality of bodies (specifically sex hormones) that plays a role in structuring women's lives needs to be addressed.

In the last three decades, feminist thinking around biology (in both its material and disciplinary senses) and its relevance to women's cultural and political positions has focused on the concepts of 'sex' and 'gender' in what has become known as 'the sex/gender debate'. At the end of the twentieth century, this debate seemed to reach a stalemate, founded, arguably, on the slipperiness of 'biology' and a failure to bring the material and disciplinary meanings of this term together in sustainable ways. Although feminist analysts had thoroughly demonstrated the cultural nature of technoscientific and biomedical discourses of biology, questions remained as to what to make of women's material differences from and similarities to men, and to each other. One important approach to this problem was to ask women to articulate their understandings and experiences of their bodies. Anthropologist Emily Martin's widely read book *The Woman in the Body: a cultural analysis of reproduction* (1987) does this in relation to hormonal bodies, studying women's conceptions and experiences of menstruation, birth and menopause and comparing and contrasting these with dominant biomedical representations of the same. Martin's study demonstrates vividly that women's relation to their bodies are both mediated by – and sometimes resist or subvert – biomedical understandings, which are themselves deeply culturally inflected.

Other debates within science and technology studies, anthropology and sociology address the question of the materiality of the body more directly, providing useful resources to overcome the stalemate within feminist theory. In particular, ethnographic studies of contemporary technoscientific and biomedical discourses demonstrate that understandings of 'the biological' or of 'life itself' are produced through embodied and culturally meaningful work. Anthropologist Sarah Franklin (2001b), for example, suggests in her work on Dolly the cloned sheep that the scientific work surrounding Dolly's birth and subsequent reproductive life demonstrates the ways in which understandings of biological life are forged through material practices of cellular manipulation, animal husbandry and breeding and scientific writing. Challenges to conventional understandings of the binary nature of mammalian sexual reproduction, Franklin argues, are literally embodied in Dolly's materiality through these practices. Such studies demonstrate that technoscientific and biomedical knowledges are not produced within cultural vacuums, but rather are the products of socio-material networks of practices and discourses.

It is vital that feminists develop ways of thinking about biology as materiality as well as, or in conjunction with, critiquing biology as a discipline. Today, women's bodies remain central to questions of power and freedom in ways that de Beauvoir could never have foreseen. Questions pertaining to sexual differences, reproduction and biological life have become increasingly pressing as biomedical and technoscientific discourses provide an ever-increasing array of explanations of, and interventions into, human and non-human bodies. Although many theorists have argued that these discourses are narrow and limiting, they do raise questions of significance for feminist and social theory: about what bodies are, how bodies are different to each other and how our experiences of ourselves are changed by technoscientific and biomedical discourses.

As for de Beauvoir, sex hormones remain at the heart of these questions today, and are hence the focus of this book. Since the early twentieth century, sex hormones have been understood as one of the key actors in producing human and non-human animal bodies and although far greater attention is currently paid to genes, hormones are thought to be central to the production of healthy, reproductive and sexually differentiated bodies. Indeed, in cutting-edge scientific fields such as proteomics and metabolomics, hormones are increasingly held to play key roles in bridging gaps between genes and bodies. As intermediaries or 'messengers' between genes and bodies, hormones feature strongly in technoscientific, biomedical *and* cultural answers to questions about sex and gender: How do foetuses develop into male and female babies? What makes boys fight and climb trees and girls play with dolls? What happens to us at puberty and where does sexual desire come from? What is a 'biological clock' and why do women (and not men?) have them? Figured as answers to such questions, sex hormones – like genes but in significantly different ways – are familiar features of contemporary western discourses on bodies. In everyday conversation and in cultural and media representations, sex hormones are understood as potent players in the production of human and non-human animal differences: we explain women's emotionalities, men's tempers and sexualities, and the reproductive desires of wild animals, our pets and ourselves, through hormones. 'Premenstrual syndrome' and 'women's moods' prior to and during menstruation, for example, are repeatedly ascribed to the action of hormones. Men's aggressive behaviour on the football pitch or in the stands is often understood as linked to testosterone. Indeed, particular public spaces such as sporting clubs or boardrooms are sometimes described as 'testosterone-soaked'. Claims regarding hormones' role in producing sexual differences and the very possibility of sexual reproduction in both humans and animals take on a more urgent character in the context of contemporary media and scientific debates over environmental oestrogens. Actors in these debates claim that hormones in the environment are changing the bodies of animals and humans with diverse effects including hastening the onset of puberty in girls and increasing infertility and reproductive-tract cancer rates across many species (see, for example, Colborn *et al.* 1996). These claims complicate understandings of hormones' role in producing sex: whilst hormones in the body are seen as central to healthy development, hormones in the environment are increasingly understood as threats to the nature of difference and life itself. As a route into critical thinking about our 'enslavement' to and 'struggle' against reproductive biologies, then, sex hormones provide fascinating case studies. The analyses of biomedical, technoscientific and cultural discourses undertaken in this book not only address specific hormone-related examples, but also explore discursive strategies for developing new lines of thought around biology, difference and 'life'. These analyses are stimulated by three key areas of social theory, introduced in the following sections: feminist theories of embodiment; science and technology (STS) theorising of non-human actors; and Foucauldian histories of biology.

Feminist theories of embodiment

The history of the sex/gender debate is one of radical, ground-breaking thought that retains a central relevance to feminist and social theory, as well as to broader cultural debate around biological aspects of life. Cultural contestations around the separation of nature and culture maintain a broad cultural prominence in the west today. Discussions of addiction, criminality, intelligence, personality and individual and familial social conditions (such as homelessness) continue to founder on the 'nature/nurture' distinction, with conservative voices claiming biological or 'natural' foundations for such behaviours or conditions. The sophistication of feminist thinking around sex and gender and the linked binary distinctions biology/culture and nature/nurture has much to offer these debates.

The use of the term gender to explain differences between men and women does not stem directly from feminist theory, but from North American research produced in the 1960s and 1970s by medical psychologists John Money and Anke Ehrhardt and psychiatrist Robert Stoller. This clinical research, developed to theorise differences deemed pathological, positioned biological sex as a structuring materiality that interacts with culture to produce gender. Gender, in this view, is connected directly, although not without cultural work, to sex. Gender, in other words, is the social interpretation of sexed biology. Following the work of de Beauvoir and responding to the naturalisation of gender differences inherent in this clinical view, feminists, in contrast, argued for a clearer distinction to be made between sex and gender. Feminist sociologist Ann Oakley (1972), for example, acknowledged biological differences between men and women, but argued that the significance of these was social. Commenting on the clinical evidence produced by Stoller and Money and colleagues, she wrote that 'The consensus of opinion seems to be that ... [biology's] role is a minimal one, in that the biological predisposition to a

male or female gender identity (if such a condition exists) may be decisively
and ineradicably overridden by cultural learning' (Oakley 1972: 170). The
note of scepticism introduced in her bracketed aside indicates the moment
in which Oakley, as a feminist sociologist, deviates from the clinical
literature. What feminists brought to debates on the sex/gender distinction
was an awareness of the *political* nature of the social production of gender
and its reliance on reference to biological sex: 'Whatever biological cause
there is in reality', Oakley writes in her concluding paragraph, 'however
influential or insubstantial it may be, thus tends to become increasingly
irrelevant and the distorted view of its importance becomes increasingly a
rationalisation of what is, in fact, only prejudice' (Oakley 1972: 210).
Unlike the clinicians, feminists did not view normative roles as healthy
or ultimately desirable, but as behaviours that (re)produced social inequi-
ties and limitations for both women and men.[1]

The understanding of gender as a social interpretation of sexed biology
was nonetheless ground-breaking and remains inspirational to much feminist and other thinking about the roles of social interpretations of biological differences. In the 1980s, however, a compelling criticism of this
position arose, informed by radical rethinkings of psychoanalysis and
poststructuralist theories. Responding to Oakley's and others' arguments,
philosophers such as Moira Gatens and Elizabeth Grosz held that the
body remains strongly significant in the production of gender. As Gatens
(1983) argued, it matters what sort of body experiences or displays gender.
Masculinity lived by a male body has very different meanings and effects to
masculinity lived by a female body. The crucial part of this position that
distinguished it from the clinical and sociological views of the intertwining
of sex and gender was its understanding of the body as itself socially
produced or inscribed. This understanding of the body, informed by
rereadings of psychoanalysis in particular, rejected a view of biology as
fixed and static, and instead posited terms such as 'morphology', 'the lived
body' and 'the imaginary body' to emphasise that although the body was
important in theorising experience, it did not dictate the content of gender
(Gatens 1983, 1996; Grosz 1989, 1990, 1994). Gatens, for example, argued
that the imaginary body is formed both by particular cultures and by
individual histories of psychical experience:

> The imaginary body is socially and historically specific in that it is constructed
> by: a shared language; the shared psychical significance and privileging of
> various zones of the body (e.g. the mouth, anus, the genitals); and the common

---

[1] See, for example, Firestone 1970; Millett 1970; Kessler and McKenna 1978.

institutional practices and discourses (e.g. medical, juridical, and educational) on and through the body.

(Gatens 1983: 152)

Positioned in between sex and gender, then, the imaginary body bridges the space between these concepts; sex and gender can no longer be seen as separable, but are also not linked in any necessary or inevitable way. Links between sex and gender are lived through the body, but are always 'socially and historically specific' in both intimate and cultural ways.

This understanding formed part of a groundswell of discussion of the body as culturally produced. In the 1980s historical texts about the body, especially medical and scientific ones, were examined in order to reveal the social nature of their descriptions.[2] Phenomenological accounts of bodily experience also emphasised the plastic and historically located nature of embodiment,[3] whilst psychoanalytic theorists wrote at length about the role of language and the unconscious in the production of bodies.[4] Michel Foucault's historical analyses of bodies within medical, scientific and legal institutions provided innovative methods and concepts for theorising the relations between bodies, knowledge and power.[5] In the 1990s, however, difficulties arose in relation to these theories of the body's cultural nature. Questions were asked as to the extent of the cultural construction of the body and about the nature of construction as a process. Although the social nature of scientific descriptions of the reproductive organs may be demonstrated (Laqueur 1992), is it possible to say how this construction constructs the flesh and blood of individual bodies? While it may be clear that phenomena such as hysterical paralysis or phantom limb indicate cultural experiences of the body (Gatens 1983; Grosz 1994), or that diet and exercise regimes produce different types of bodies (Bordo 1993; Gatens 1996: 68–9), what of less visible, microscopic body elements such as chromosomes, and indeed hormones? Are they culturally constructed? Do they exist outside of representations of them and, if so, how can we gain any access to this? If descriptions are always social, does this necessarily mean that bodies are entirely social too?

In feminist theory these questions coalesced in the late 1980s and early 1990s around the issue of essentialism and how to understand differences between the sexes. Questions about the cultural construction of the body led feminists to ask what the nature of difference actually was. If some

---

[2] See, for example, Gallagher and Laqueur 1987; Schiebinger 1989; Laqueur 1992.
[3] See, for example, Young 1990; Duden 1991, 1993; Bordo 1993.
[4] See, for example, Kristeva 1982; Irigaray 1985, 1993b; Grosz 1989; de Lauretis 1994.
[5] Foucault 1987, 1988, 1994, 1995.

difference was to be claimed between men and women in terms of embodiment, what did this rely on? Was some sort of biological claim being made (thereby making the argument essentialist) or, on the other hand, was an impossibly flexible body being posited in which all differences were social and changeable? These debates caused a crisis in feminist theory as they led to the questioning of the status of the category 'women' itself. If there was no essential (biological or otherwise) commonality between women, could they be considered a group? These debates were also fuelled by the research and political interventions of Black and anti-racist feminists and lesbian and queer theorists who criticised the racist and heterosexist understandings of the term 'women' prevalent in much feminist theory.[6]

The strengthening and reworking of the term 'gender' has been one major response to this dilemma. Central to this response is the work of Judith Butler and the various interpretations of it made by queer and feminist theorists. The 1990 publication of *Gender Trouble* and the development of its argument in *Bodies that Matter* (1993) and *Undoing Gender* (2004) have had an enormous impact on the status of the word 'gender' and its relation to 'sex' and 'the body'. In all these books Butler makes a complex argument about the cultural production of both gender and sex and how this creates what we understand to be sexed embodiment. She argues that the construction of gendered and sexed experience takes place through a lifetime of repeated performative acts. For Butler, neither sex nor gender is 'natural': both are produced as effects of iterated actions that are culturally intelligible. She argues that the prevalent conceptualisation of two 'natural' sexes is produced through the operation of gender to read as if the operation works in the opposite direction (that gender stems from sex). Sex and sexed bodies, in other words, materialise through the operation of gender, an operation that is itself obscured.

The notion of repeated performative acts constituting gender is not about willed action; Butler wants to capture some of the relative inescapability of culturally produced gender (Butler 1993: 12–16, 94–5; 1994). Gender, she argues, is produced within particular cultural constraints – a 'matrix of schemas' – that although not fixed throughout time, are not easy to resist. In fact, she argues, these constraints are *necessary* to the production of gender: the performative acts constituting gender cannot be understood outside the constrained repetition of cultural norms and conventions (Butler 1993: 94–5). Developing Foucault's thesis in the *History of*

---

[6] See, for example, Riley 1988; hooks 1990; Sedgwick 1991; Butler 1993; Gunew and Yeatman 1993; Hammonds 1994; Rubin 1994; Wiegman 1995.

Sexuality: an introduction regarding the operation of power through the establishment of norms, Butler writes:

> 'Sex' is always produced as a reiteration of hegemonic norms. This productive reiteration can be read as a kind of performativity ... [H]owever, this productive capacity of discourses is derivative, a form of cultural iterability, a practice of *re*signification, not a creation ex nihilo ... [P]erformatives constitute a locus of discursive production. No 'act' apart from a regularized and sanctioned practice can wield the power to produce that which it declares. Indeed, a performative act apart from a reiterated and hence sanctioned set of conventions can appear only as vain effort to produce effects that it cannot possibly produce.
>
> *(Butler 1993: 107, emphasis in original)*

The norms of gender, in other words, constitute limits to culturally intelligible actions and existence. When people act in ways that do not reproduce norms they 'risk internment and imprisonment', are liable to be subjected to violence and to become 'criminalized and pathologized' (Butler 2004: 30). Indeed, in her most recent work Butler argues that these norms of gender have significance for the most basic level of existence: 'The normative aspiration at work here has to do with the ability to live and breathe and move' (Butler 2004: 31).

For Butler, then, norms *materialise* bodies and sex. As an alternative to essentialism or the positing of a stable or basic matter (sex or biology), which is then worked on by culture (gender), Butler proposes 'a return to the notion of matter, not as a site or surface, but as *a process of materialization that stabilizes over time to produce the effect of boundary, fixity, and surface we call matter*' (Butler 1993: 9, emphasis in original). In this concept of materialisation Butler refuses a linguistic monism that posits all materiality as an effect of language, relying instead on a Foucauldian notion of the productive nature of regulatory power. Despite this, she stresses her desire to refuse any 'concession' to the materiality of the body, or the undeniability of the differences between the sexes (although she says that when questioned she inevitably makes such concessions), because she believes there can be no access to materiality except through language or discourse. It is important to note here, however, that Butler argues that this statement is different from suggesting that discourse is responsible for the creation of everything or 'that it originates, causes, or exhaustively composes that which it concedes' (Butler 1993: 10). It is to claim, rather, that 'There is no reference to a pure body which is not at the same time a further formation of that body' (Butler 1993: 10).

Despite the convincing nature of these arguments, the *extent* of this materialisation of sex and the body remains unclear. As philosopher Pheng Cheah (1996) argues, Butler ends up making a distinction between the production or materialisation of the outlines or boundaries of the body and the production of the actual materiality of biological processes. Although Butler emphasises the role of language in the production of what she calls the morphological body, she *is* forced to make some concession regarding biological processes such as endocrinological systems. Whilst it is clear that discourse shapes our understanding of and relation to these processes, it is another thing to argue that discourse or the repetition of norms *produces* them. As Butler writes:

> Here the materiality of the body ought not to be conceptualised as a unilateral or causal *effect* of the psyche in any sense that would reduce that materiality to the psyche or make of the psyche the monistic stuff out of which that materiality is produced and/or derived. This latter alternative would constitute a clearly untenable form of idealism. It must be possible to concede and affirm an array of 'materialities' that pertain to the body, that which is signified by the domains of biology, anatomy, physiology, hormonal and chemical composition, illness, weight, metabolism, life and death. None of this can be denied.
>
> *(Butler 1993: 66)*

However, as discussed above, Butler argues convincingly that there can be no access to this materiality unstructured by cultural discourses (especially those around sexual difference) and that these materialities can therefore never be used as unadulterated grounds for political claims. That materialities cannot be denied does not mean, she maintains, that they can ever simply be affirmed:

> But the undeniability of these 'materialities' in no way implies what it means to affirm them, indeed, what interpretive matrices condition, enable and limit that necessary affirmation. That each of these categories have a history and a historicity, that each of them is constituted through the boundary lines that distinguish them and, hence, by what they exclude, that relations of discourse and power produce hierarchies and overlappings among them and challenge those boundaries, implies that these are *both* persistent and contested regions.
>
> *(Butler 1993: 67, emphasis in original)*

Whilst this distinction between affirmation and the impossibility of denial is small, it is nonetheless theoretically significant. It provides a route into addressing the distinction raised earlier between biology as a discipline and as materiality. Although, following Butler, we cannot approach materiality in any direct way, it does not therefore become necessary to deny that biological actors exist and may have effects.[7]

---

[7] Despite these comments, Cheah (1996) convincingly argues that Butler tends to focus in *Gender Trouble* and *Bodies That Matter* on social and psychical rather than biological

For sex hormones, which seem to be entities whose materiality cannot be denied, this form of argument is highly pertinent. Although to deny the existence of hormones is difficult (and arguably politically inadvisable), it would be equally inadvisable and incorrect to accept any knowledge or speaking about hormones as simply true or reflective of their materiality. 'Biology' or 'materiality' (and terms like 'hormones' that occupy the same domain) may be terms like 'women' that, despite their difficulties, should not be discarded. As Butler argues regarding the use of 'women' in feminist politics, the point is to examine carefully the use of any term, not to reject it. 'I would like to raise the question of whether recourse to matter and to the materiality of sex is necessary in order to establish that irreducible specificity that is said to ground feminist practice', she writes,

> and here the question is not whether or not there ought to be reference to matter, just as the question never has been whether or not there ought to be speaking about women. This speaking will occur, and for feminist reasons, it must; the category of women does not become useless through deconstruction, but becomes one whose uses are no longer reified as 'referents', and which stand a chance of being opened up, indeed, of coming to signify in ways that none of us can predict in advance. Surely, it must be possible both to use the term, to use it tactically even as one is, as it were, used and positioned by it, and also to subject the term to a critique which interrogates the exclusionary operations and differential power relations that construct and delimit feminist invocations of 'women'.
>
> *(Butler 1993: 29)*

Butler's deconstructionist position in relation to the terms 'women' and 'matter' has remained opaque to many who are inspired by her work on gender. Some queer theorists and feminists re-cite Butler's theories in ways that fail to recognise the centrality of Spivak's (1994) point about deconstruction cited by Butler following the above quotation: deconstruction is the critique of something useful, that we cannot do without. These theorists instead tend towards arguing that sex is something that we *can* do without – that all that is important is a concept of gender premised on its

---

forces. Her understanding of the dynamism of matter is unnecessarily restricted to human bodies through her focus on the role of psychical identification with images or schemas in the production of subjectivity and embodiment. This type of understanding makes too great a distinction between human and non-human – a distinction that is problematic in its political and practical effects on the lives and existence of both humans and non-humans, especially because it tends to posit the non-human world as passive. Cheah suggests that Butler's focus on the discursive constraints on the materialisation of bodies means that '[S]he has little to say about scenarios of contestation where the constraints on and enabling conditions for the resignification of identity are primarily material rather than discursive, economic rather than ideational' (Cheah 1996: 134).

fluidity and flexibility. This type of argument has the effect, Butler (1994) argues, of denying the importance of sexual difference, especially in relation to studies of sexuality, and of hiding from view the contested history of the sex/gender distinction.

In the mid-1990s, feminist theorist Biddy Martin also noted this tendency, arguing that some queer theorists tended to position gender as inherently negative. Celebrating fluid sexuality and radical performativity, queer theorists and the popular queer press of the time, Martin suggested, positioned feminism as 'anachronistic' and 'superseded' in its (supposed) focus on gender (Martin 1996: 71). This negative view of gender became linked with femininity and the female body through its association with feminism. Although she recognised its great value, Martin claimed that

> lesbian and gay work fails at times to realize its potential for reconceptualizing the complexities of identity and social relations, at moments when, almost in spite of itself, it at least implicitly conceives gender in negative terms, in the terms of fixity, miring, or subjection to the indicatively female body, with the consequence that escape from gender, usually in the form of disembodiment and always in the form of gender crossings, becomes the goal and the putative achievement.
>
> *(Martin 1996: 73)*

This was especially evident, Martin argues, in queer theories' relation to femme lesbians, who were figured as caught in this ensnaring femininity (femininity performed parodically in drag, for example, was okay; femininity 'played straight' in everyday life was not).[8]

Martin applauds Butler's attention to the materiality of the body but suggests that the criticism sometimes made that Butler's work 'fail[s] at times to make the body enough of a drag on signification' is partially correct (Martin 1996: 80). 'In the effort to highlight obvious sexual differences and defiances of norms', she suggests, 'that all-too-obvious and thus invisible difference that it makes to be a woman drops out of view' (Martin 1996: 82). Thus with regard to the popular documentary film *Paris is Burning* discussed by Butler, in which cross-dressing, preoperative

---

[8] Martin also suggests that an exclusive focus on socially produced and flexible gender and an exclusion of any consideration of interiority or psychical life (beyond that which is seen as the result of normalisation) can 'impoverish the language we have available for thinking about selves and relationships, even as they apparently enrich our vocabularies for thinking about social construction' (Martin 1996: 174). A focus on exteriority and the reduction of subjectivities to effects of power can position psychical life as fixed or passive in the same way that the body is so positioned in some theorisations of gender. Again Martin sees a connection with a limiting view of the feminine and the female body, as interiority is aligned with a negative, fixed femininity.

transsexual sex worker Venus Xtravaganza is murdered by a client, Martin argues that two interpretations are available. One is certainly the interpretation that Butler offers: that the male client thought Venus was a woman and killed him/her when he realised s/he had a penis. But there is also another possibility. Venus may have been murdered because (or whilst) the client thought she was a woman. To suggest only the first option, Martin contends, is to focus too exclusively on radical cross-gender performance and to render invisible the violence that women often receive in everyday life.[9] These two options are further complicated by the potential operation of racism in this case. Venus Xtravaganza was Black, a fact that, as Butler suggests, has significance for understanding his/her murder. Whichever of the two versions is more accurate – that s/he was murdered by someone who thought s/he was a woman or who realised s/he had a penis – racism could have fuelled the hatred leading to his/her death.

Butler and Martin agree, then, that a focus on gender at the expense of sex and sexual difference can mean a belittling of the importance of race and class issues (Butler 1994: 15–16; Martin 1996: 73). A refocusing on the body and the 'drag' of its materiality can help here. If this drag is acknowledged (although, as Martin stresses, this drag cannot be predetermined in shape or content) then differences relating to sexual difference, race and class can be accounted for. Although we might not want to ascribe any particular ahistorical content to sexual difference, race or class, it is important not to diminish their effects through a positing of excessive flexibility. As Martin writes, 'too little emphasis on the difference it [the drag of the body] makes risks the elimination of difference in a kind of postmodern humanism of (im)possibility' (Martin 1996: 92). The question of historicity is also central here, and the importance of the longevity of social structures and discourses about various differences and resistances to them must not be underestimated. 'When it comes to questions of gender, sexuality, and identity, however', Martin writes,

---

[9] This issue comes up in Butler's more recent work. In a chapter on 'Gender Regulations' in *Undoing Gender*, for example, she writes about the 'social punishments that follow upon trangressions of gender' performed by intersexed, transsexed, transgendered and 'gender dysphoric' or 'gender-troubled' people (Butler 2004: 55). This focus shares a tendency with the story about Venus Xtravaganza to sideline the (albeit substantially different) suffering experienced by those who perform normative gender well, particularly heterosexual women. Performing non-normative gender is certainly highly risky, but performing normative gender has serious negative implications for women also.

temporality reminds us that inside/outside encounters have the effect again and again of making bodies and psyches with histories that then exert their own pressures back on the boundaries between out and in, back on what we take to be the social world around a self or a person. Though that body and psyche can be said to be effects of power, they are irreducible to it. Though never constituted outside of given social/discursive relations, power also moves from bodies/psyches/minds outward, not by virtue of will, but by virtue of the pressure exerted by what's given in the form of body and subjectivity.

(Martin 1996: 93)

In *Undoing Gender*, Butler comes closer than in the two earlier books to Martin's understanding of the body as something that drags or 'exerts pressure'. Engaging with the work of activists in the intersex movement, for example, Butler makes stronger claims that the norms of gender both stretch towards, but are also resisted by, the actual life of a body (meaning both 'the minimal biological form of living' and 'the minimal conditions for a liveable life with regard to human life') (Butler 2004: 226). The writing of intersex activists shows both that the effects of gender norms are profound and consequential for those who live outside them and that some people have always, and will always, live outside these norms. The aim of feminist theory and politics, then, is to develop 'a new legitimating lexicon for the gender complexity that we have always been living' (Butler 2004: 219). In Martin's terms we could understand this as the pressure exerted back on the world by intersexed bodies: although in many senses vulnerable, such bodies and lives are not reducible to the effects of psychiatric and biomedical power that defines them as pathological. If we understand intersexuality as linked to hormonal specificities, this pressure or drag needs to be thought at the endocrinological level, albeit without reducing intersexuality to simply a biological phenomenon.[10]

Although Martin (1996: 92) refers to the materiality of the body as both a potential and a limit, there is a tendency in her work and in the work of Butler to focus on materiality as constraint (the word 'drag' suggests this). Other feminist theorists, inspired by the work of philosophers Gilles Deleuze and Felix Guattari, describe the materiality of the body in more positive terms. In her book *Time Travels: feminism, nature, power*, for example, Elizabeth Grosz (2005: 44) talks of 'the biological forces that press on and produce life'. Whilst this is very close to Martin's 'pressure of what's given', Grosz specifically argues against the notion that biological forces (which she sometimes calls 'the natural') constrain culture.

---

[10] The hormonal aspects of intersexuality are discussed in Chapter 2.

.'The natural does not limit the cultural', she writes, 'it provokes and incites the cultural by generating problems, questions, events that must be addressed and negotiated, symbolized, or left unrepresented' (Grosz 2005: 51).[11] Feminist philosopher Rosi Braidotti makes a similar claim about the productivity of vital forces, but does this through distinguishing two understandings of biology: *zoe* ('the generative vitality of non- or pre-human or animal life') and *bios* (human life that is immersed in politics and discourse) (Braidotti 2006: 37). Her work focuses on exploring the positive and repressed role of *zoe* in contemporary life, an exploration that 'refers to the endless vitality of life as continuous becoming' (Braidotti 2006: 41), as well as understanding the multiple ways in which bio- and other technologies work with bodies as *bios*. Theorised in relational combination, *bios* and *zoe*, Braidotti writes,

> create an unexpected form of contiguity between material processes of constitution of areas or objects of interest, like the 'cell', or the 'seed' and processes of subjectivation. In other words, it is not that 'life' is being vampirized by bio-technology but rather that, as a result of bio-technological material and discursive practices, 'life as *bios/zoe*' produces ever-growing new areas of activity and intervention.
>
> *(Braidotti 2006: 55)*

Despite their insistence on the significance of vital biological forces, however, neither Grosz nor Braidotti discuss detailed examples of these. In contrast, my aim in this book is to analyse sex hormones as a way to address questions of materiality and the sexed biological body in more fine-grained detail. Engaging both with endogenous hormones (those generated by the body with no medical intervention and that seem to be necessary for human and other animal lives) and with hormones taken as medicine (often based on the endogenous hormones of other species such as horses or rodents) or encountered in the external environment, this book theorises hormones as a form of pressure exerted on the world (to use Martin's phrase) that is productive and yet co-produced with normative technoscientific and biomedical discourses.

---

[11] This position is in some ways a departure from Grosz's earlier work in *Volatile Bodies* (1994), in which the biological was understood as a limit on culture. This work is discussed in more detail in Chapter 3. In her recent work, Grosz also positions her argument in direct contradiction to Butler's theories of performativity. Like Cheah, Grosz criticises Butler for focusing only on the dynamism of human forces in the production of subjectivity. In *Time Travels*, Grosz argues that non-human forces must also be theorised as active in the production of sexed subjects (Grosz 2005: 189–90).

Science studies and the active body

A contemporary stream of thinking in science and technology studies that attempts to understand non-human and non-living objects as active in the construction of worlds provides important direction in this book's endeavours. Deriving from the work of Bruno Latour, Steve Woolgar, Michael Callon, John Law and others from the late 1970s to the present, this approach reads science and technology from a sociological perspective that acknowledges the power of scientific practice but does not accept a traditional view of science as objective and detached knowledge. It emphasises the importance of moving beyond an analysis of the social context of science and technology, towards analysing their content; in fact, Latour (1988) postulates that the distinction between 'science' and 'society' is untenable. Importantly, the 'content' of science refers here to a set of practices or meaning-making work. In their early analysis of a neuro-endocrinology laboratory, for example, Latour and Woolgar wrote:

> Our claim is not just that TRF [a hormone] is surrounded, influenced by, in part depends on, or is also caused by circumstances; rather, we argue that science is entirely fabricated out of circumstance; moreover, it is precisely through specific localised practices that science appears to escape all circumstances.
> *(Latour and Woolgar 1979: 239)*

This actor-network theory (ANT) approach to the analysis of science makes a radical shift in the understanding of science's objects.[12] Instead of following the traditional view that positions the scientist as subject and whatever he or she is studying as object (a view that has also been strongly critiqued by feminists), an ANT approach posits every player in the story of scientific work as an actor. This includes scientists and technicians, funding bodies, other groups of people affected, the apparatus used and any living or non-living entity involved (such as insects, microbes, hormones and chemicals). An understanding of the processes of science is then formed through a detailed analysis of the interactions of all of these actors, of how the actors combine and interact in order to achieve what is best for them.[13]

---

[12] This shift took place in Latour's later works, rather than in his and Woolgar's 1979 *Laboratory Life*, although many of the notions Latour relies on later were developed in this earlier ground-breaking book. Callon's work, although it has its differences from Latour's, makes very similar points regarding the activity of the objects of science (Callon 1986; see also Martin 1995).

[13] As is discussed in Chapter 1, this view of science as a competition or battle where each actor struggles to achieve its own ends has been criticised by some feminists as masculinist and Machiavellian (see Haraway 1989: 6, and 1991: 185–6; Amsterdamska 1990; Winner 1993).

Actors such as microbes or particular hormones are not, Latour specifies, 'natural' agents that are discovered by science (Latour 1988: 107). Rather they are entities that exist for a certain time within a network of forces and practices that allow them to flourish – they are allies in the scientific process. If an entity is proposed that does more, that allows better claims to be made, the older one will become redundant. In scientific literature, however, the operations of science are represented as being about the existence of natural entities, about the discovery of facts. By this representation, Latour argues, the processes of the enlistment of allies to produce certain scientific understandings and practices are obscured and the allies of scientists are made to appear as passive objects.

Although there are limitations to the ANT approach, the emphasis on the active nature of all entities involved in science is ground-breaking and useful. In the attempt to understand hormones as active entities, it is helpful to see them as allies of particular worldviews, rather than as naturally occurring objects 'discovered' by science. However, as is pointed out by science studies theorist Olga Amsterdamska (1990), it is important not to ignore the differences between human and non-human actors in science (as she accuses Latour of doing). As Amsterdamska (1990: 501) argues, 'the goals, the means, and the results of enrolling such different kinds of "allies" are hardly comparable, and that the elimination of differences among them leads only to confusion'. Emily Martin makes a similar point, arguing that Latour and Callon only allow for the activity of non-human actors insofar as these actors can be said to compete in the same way as human actors (as 'accumulating entrepreneur[s]') and that this negates differences between human and non-human actors (Martin 1995: 267). Unless the differences between actors, allies and the methods used to enlist them in a scientific process are acknowledged, no political or ethical claims can be made about these processes and their effects (although, again, it is important not to assume the nature of these differences or to ascribe them any ahistorical content).

The notion of the activity of non-human actors in science has been taken up and reworked by a number of feminist science-studies theorists including Susan Leigh Star (1991), Nelly Oudshoorn (1994; 2003), Annemarie Mol (2002) and others (Mol and Law 1994; Mol and Mesman 1996) and Adele Clarke and Joan Fugimura (1992). The work of North American science-studies theorist Donna Haraway (1978, 1989, 1991, 1992a, 1992b, 1997, 2003) is exemplary in this regard. Like Latour, Haraway argues that science is better understood if its objects – the world or nature – are seen not only as cultural, but also as active. Her version of

the activity of nature, however, avoids the problems brought up by
Amsterdamska and Martin's critique of Latour by stressing the distinction
between activity and agency (described in a footnote as a distinction
between the terms 'actors' and 'actants') (Haraway 1992a: 331). She argues
that nature and all the entities involved in science are active, but not
necessarily in a way that implies human-like agency or character (as the
term 'actor' implies). Haraway's preference is for the word 'actant' because
it implies something that is active at the level of function rather than
identity; it allows for differences between humans and non-humans
(machines, animals and others) that can then be understood as active
without being anthropomorphised. Haraway theorises nature as 'coyote'
or as a coding trickster, as made up of various historically specific (time-
and place-specific) combinations of actants – a theorising that talks about
activity without relying on liberal theories of identity and agency
(Haraway 1991: 199; 1992b: 331). She describes these combining practices
as articulated through story-telling, arguing that science and all other
knowledges produce stories about the world in combination with different
actants: 'Worldly and enspirited, coyote nature is a collective, cosmopol-
itan artifact crafted in stories with heterogenous actants' (Haraway 1992b:
332). What Haraway is interested in politically is examining how these
stories produce worlds and how other stories can be told that produce less
exploitative situations for all beings. 'If the world exists for us as "nature"',
she writes,

> this designates a kind of relationship, an achievement among many actors, not
> all of them human, not all of them organic, not all of them technological. In
> its scientific embodiments as well as in other forms, nature is made, but not
> entirely by humans; it is a co-construction among humans and non-humans.
>
> *(Haraway 1992b: 297)*

Haraway's understanding of bodies is underpinned by this argument
about the relational co-production of nature. Like Butler, Haraway takes
a position that rejects both a biological determinist argument and one that
understands bodies as entirely cultural ideological productions. She
argues, again like Butler, that there can be no access to bodies outside of
language or discourse ('Biology is a discourse, not the living world itself'),
but that this does not mean that language forms bodies (Haraway 1992b:
298). Referring to her well-known formulation of bodies as 'material-
semiotic actors' (Haraway 1991: 200), Haraway emphasises that this
phrase was meant to stress the importance of the object of knowledge in
the production of bodies, 'without *ever* implying the immediate presence of
such objects or, what is the same thing, their final or unique determination

of what can count as objective knowledge of a biological body at a particular historical juncture' (Haraway 1992b: 298). Thus she argues that bodies, like nature in general, materialise in social interaction between human and non-human actors and actants. These materialisations occur within structures of power and knowledge including scientific journals, cultural images and texts, visual technologies and all types of research. Entities such as hormones and the endocrinological system, then, are constructs of elaborate systems of knowledge and power, but are also active – they are not fantasies, but materialisations that have enormous effects on embodiments and lives (Haraway 1992b: 298).

For me, Haraway's approach to bodies opens up space for theorising hormones as active in the ongoing materialisation of sex and sexual difference. Understanding hormones as material-semiotic actors means that their activities can be analysed without alignment with biological determinism. If hormones are material-semiotic actors, questions about their role in the production of sexual difference change. Rather than asking, as does psychiatrist Simon Baron-Cohen (2004: 96) in his popular book *The Essential Difference*, 'Can biology account for ... sex differences?' *Messengers of Sex* asks, 'How are sex hormones figured in technoscientific and biomedical accounts of sex differences, and how might we theorise their material-semiotic role in combination with – rather than in opposition to – sociocultural factors like language and social norms?' In contrast to the questions posed by Baron-Cohen and the other technoscientific, biomedical and popular literatures analysed in this book, these questions neither reproduce conceptual divisions between 'the social' and 'the biological' nor affirm the importance of either against their so-called opposite. Rather, they investigate and ultimately disrupt these historically significant categories.

Foucault's histories of bodies

Michel Foucault's historical analyses provide the third stimulus for my analysis of sex hormones and questions pertaining to biological life. If questions of power are obscured in actor-network-theory approaches to technoscience and biomedicine, Foucault's histories of biomedicine (especially his work on madness and sexuality) constitute important antidotes.

In *The History of Sexuality: an introduction*, Foucault discusses how his research addresses the biological body, and calls for a 'history of bodies', rather than a history of thought about the body. He begins by posing a question, 'First, does the analysis of sexuality necessarily imply the elision of the body, anatomy, the biological, the functional?', and responds:

> To this question, I think we can reply in the negative. In any case, the purpose of the present study is in fact to show how deployments of power are directly connected to the body – to bodies, functions, physiological processes, sensations, and pleasures; far from the body having to be effaced, what is needed is to make it visible through an analysis in which the biological and the historical are not consecutive to one another, as in the evolutionism of the first sociologists, but are bound together in an increasingly complex fashion in accordance with the development of the modern technologies of power that take life as their objective. Hence I do not envisage a 'history of mentalities' that would take account of bodies only through the manner in which they have been perceived and given meaning and value; but a 'history of bodies' and the manner in which what is most material and most vital in them has been invested.
>
> *(Foucault 1987: 151–2)*

Foucault's call, like that of Haraway, is to focus on bodies themselves – what is 'most vital in them' – rather than to assume that bodies are natural and precede sociality. In this history, Foucault names the 'modern technologies of power' that 'are directly connected to the body – to bodies, functions, physiological processes, sensations, and pleasures', *biopower* (Foucault 1987: 143). Biopower, he argues, is a new form of power that takes hold of material bodies and organises them as living organisms. Biopower organises the social by regulating the activities and 'nature' of bodies at both individual and population levels through the production of scientific and medical discourses that observe, measure and act upon bodies.

Although Foucault's discussion of biopower is only brief, the concept is widely used in social scientific analyses of contemporary biomedicine and technoscience. Anthropologist Paul Rabinow (1992), for example, offers the term 'biosociality' as an elaboration of biopower that speaks specifically to late twentieth-century biomedicine. In a biosocial world, Rabinow suggests, biomedical and technoscientific discourses produce subjects whose sociality clusters around biomedical categories: we understand ourselves as belonging to groups of people who share similar genetic propensities or diseases or whose children suffer from particular medical conditions. Sociologist Nikolas Rose (2001) develops a related argument, suggesting that in the later part of the twentieth century, biopower as described by Foucault changed – rather than a system of power implying a gap between 'those who calculated and exercised power and those who were its subjects', biopower became 'democratised' (Rose 2001: 17). This democratisation occurred through the alignment of governmental desires for a healthy population with individual aspirations for life fulfilment, at both psychological and biological levels. 'By the start of the 21st century', then, Rose suggests,

> hopes, fears, decisions and life-routines shared in terms of the risks and possibilities in corporeal and biological existence had come to supplant almost all others as organizing principles of a life of prudence, responsibility and choice.
>
> *(Rose 2001: 18)*

This move towards personal responsibility for health and biological futures, Rose argues, is also aligned with an expansion of what has become known as bioeconomics: the circulation of elements of human and non-human biologies as products within global economies (see also Novas and Rose 2000; Waldby 2000).

Focault's focus on the genealogical aspects of contemporary aspects of biology and biomedicine is of great importance to my argument here. Throughout this book, I use the term bio-social to describe the contemporary situation analysed by Rabinow and Rose. My insertion of a hyphen signals a small departure from their analyses, however; namely, a desire to insist that the implosion of the biological and the social is not as advanced or wide-ranging as their work sometimes implies. As in Haraway's 'material-semiotic', the hyphen in bio-social signals an important tension that, as I will demonstrate throughout *Messengers of Sex*, remains very much in play in the multiple fields of hormone messaging. The hyphen, in other words, marks a space for the messaging activities themselves.

Messaging sex

The word 'hormone' comes from the Greek word *hormao* meaning 'I excite, arouse' or 'put into quick action'. Hormones have been understood through the twentieth century as chemicals that not only arouse or excite particular physical reactions, behaviours or emotions, but also sexual difference itself; within biomedical and technoscientific discourses, hormones are seen as 'messengers of sex'. Although common, this phrase is never unpacked, thus leaving many interesting and important questions unasked: for example, if hormones are messengers of sex, what is the message? And to whom is the message sent? Is it from one part of the body to another or from the body to the world? Analysing the history of endocrinology in Part I, and contemporary textbooks and scientific papers describing the actions of hormones in Part II, I argue that the common implication of this phrase is that hormones carry a message of sex from one part of the body to another, exciting or arousing a physical expression of inherent (genetic) sex. Sex hormones, in other words, operate within (relatively) closed biological or bodily systems, carrying messages that stimulate cells to produce proteins that act to create sexed brains, organs, bodies and behaviours. In this conventional technoscientific sense, hormones are messengers *of* sex in the sense both that they derive *from* (inherent) sex and that they *lead to* the creation of, or produce (material) sex.

Messengers of Sex argues for a refigured view of hormones as messengers of sex, suggesting that hormones do not message an inherent or preexisting sex within bodies, but rather are active agents in bio-social systems that constitute material-semiotic entities known as 'sex'. This view follows from the feminist and critical science studies debates outlined above and allows for a particular intervention into feminist debates about 'gender', 'women' and 'sex'. Whilst hormones may well be one bodily messenger of difference between what we name as 'the sexes', this does not mean that sexual difference and/or gender is *produced* or constituted by hormones. As described in Chapters 1 and 2, hormones are chemicals that exist in differential amounts in different bodies, producing significant effects on these bodies. The existence of certain ratios of different hormones in bodies is not random, but follows strong patterns across vast numbers of humans and other species and if these patterns are greatly diverged from in any particular individual, the effects on that individual's body are usually quite stark (for example, the person or animal may not develop gonads or reproductive organs that fit within a statistically normal range or that can participate in sexual reproduction). But hormones also exist outside of bodies in the form of environmental toxins, as is discussed in Chapter 6. These hormones (and other chemicals that act like hormones) enter bodies and interact with endocrine systems. The actions of hormones can also not be understood outside of cultural descriptions of these actions and of 'sex' itself.

The argument of *Messengers of Sex*, then, is that while hormones may excite or provoke sexual difference through their effects on bodies, they neither simply express nor produce sex.[14] Hormones' messaging is received and responded to within bio-social (as opposed to purely biological)

---

[14] This argument may be compared to Butler's description of the anatomical body as demand; as something both caught up in systems of signification (and which can only be understood through these) and which exceeds that signification. Butler writes:

> The anatomical is only 'given' through its signification, and yet it appears to exceed that signification, to provide the elusive referent in relation to which the variability of signification performs. Always already caught up in the signifying chain by which

systems or worlds. Sexually differentiated bodies are produced and understood within cultures that precede any individual and that are constantly giving meanings to differences, and hormones always perform their messaging activity within cultures. Although their actions are not limited to representation, just as sex or the body is not limited to (social) gender, we can only understand them in socio-cultural terms. These socio-cultural terms are historically specific (although some of them last for very long periods of time) and are therefore contestable. It is the role of feminist work to produce critical analyses of existing formulations of these actions *and* to develop new concepts and frameworks for understanding and influencing the bio-social activity of actors like hormones.

This view of hormones may prove of use both theoretically and politically to feminism, especially insofar as it can be extended to considerations of biology more generally. As Butler (1993), Spivak with Rooney (1994) and others argue, it is important for feminism not to abandon words like 'women' and 'biology' in an attempt to achieve theoretical purity. These are words that feminism cannot do without. How, for example, could feminists intervene in debates around the politics of hormonal medications such as the pill and hormone-replacement therapy, if we refused to talk about biology and spoke only of gender? At a political level, such a move would only ensure a lack of attention being given to our interventions. But this is not to argue for merely a 'strategic' use of biology and sex. For, as argued above, there are strong theoretical arguments against the notion that 'everything is social', that everything to do with women can be understood through an analysis of gender. If we grant activity to entities other than human subjectivities, we must accept this. To fail to do so is to place humans above all other entities, including the living and non-living, and to position the non-human world as passive. This can only mean an impoverished and unconvincing understanding of the world that would limit our ability to generate change. Reading hormones or biology as a provocation to the social is a way of understanding

> sexual difference is negotiated, the anatomical is never outside its terms, and yet it is also that which exceeds and compels that signifying chain, that reiteration of difference, an insistent and inexhaustible demand.
>
> *(Butler 1993: 90)*

The main difference between this notion of the anatomical body as demand and my proposal of biology as provocation is the emphasis Butler gives to the role of language and signification that, as Cheah (1996) suggests, limits her observations to the human realm. The notion of biology as provocation is intended to move beyond this limit in its emphasis on the activity of the biological.

them as a 'drag' on the productive power of culture that is not static and negative (as Martin argued sex becomes in some queer arguments), but that allows for the activity and changeability of the world, the body and nature. It reads the history of nature and sex without reducing them to histories of representation, because the body or nature is active, rather than a passive, unchanging essence. As Foucault's work suggests, such an approach facilitates 'a "history of bodies" and the manner in which what is most material and most vital in them has been invested' (Foucault 1987: 152; see also Gatens 1996: 60–75).

Organisation of the book

This book is interdisciplinary in scope. The selection of materials for analysis is in some ways eclectic, for interdisciplinary work cannot cover material produced in every social scientific and humanist discipline. Similarly, critical work on science, medicine and technology cannot engage in equal depth with every scientific, medical or technical discipline. Interdisciplinary work must, in other words, be selective. The materials in this book come from the following disciplines: history, philosophy, science and technology studies, cultural studies, anthropology and sociology. Whilst it would be valid to discuss literature from linguistics, media studies, nursing and literary theory, amongst other disciplines, materials from these fields are only rarely included here. Theoretical and methodological approaches developed in the interdisciplinary field of women's studies underpin the analysis of all these materials. The scientific, medical and technical materials examined here come from physiology, biology, behavioural endocrinology, psychology, endocrinology, sexology, gerontology and environmental toxicology. The selection of these disciplines is less eclectic: these are the fields that deal in most detail with developing explanations of the action of hormones in sexually differentiated bodies.

Messengers of Sex is divided into three parts. The first, 'Hormone histories', examines the history of sex, investigating the coming-into-being of the hormonally sexed body in late nineteenth and early twentieth-century Europe. This chapter describes how hormones came to be understood as central to the development of sexual differences in humans. It shows how the suggestion of hormones as messengers was transmuted into strong medical and scientific claims about sex hormones' role in producing what feminist science-studies theorist Nelly Oudshoorn (1994) has called 'the hormonal body'.

Part II, 'Hormonal bodies', focuses on contemporary technoscientific understandings of hormones' role in the production of sexed bodies and behaviours. Examining physiology, biology, psychology and behavioural endocrinology, the chapters critically discuss the biological/social distinction. Bringing critical scientists' work on the responsiveness of the biological to the social together with feminist theories of the body and discussions of essentialism, I argue for a rethinking of this distinction. Haraway's notion of articulation provides an alternative way of thinking through science's relation to biology as materiality.

Part III, 'Hormone cultures', addresses the movement of sex hormones into bodies as medications and in accidental or environmental events. In both cases, the focus is on cultural understandings of the role of exogenous sex hormones in producing sexual differences. Chapters 4 and 5 address the development and contemporary use of hormone-replacement therapies for both men and women. I examine the production of specific and limiting versions of sexual differences through the use of hormones and argue that these productions are interwoven with particular understandings of class and racial differences. Chapter 6 turns to hormones in the environment and scientific and popular discourses around their impact on the production of sexually differentiated human bodies. All of the chapters in this Part document the movement of hormones into bodies and explore how these actions can be theorised without recourse to biological determinism.

Each Part investigates the nature of the hormonally sexed body: its history and production within technoscience; its technologisation in contemporary biomedicine; and its position within today's changing environments. As discussed above, the aim of these investigations is not to dismiss or affirm the biological, but rather to demonstrate its complexity and its interwovenness with the social. My goal is to produce work that will be valuable to women's and gender studies, science studies and social theory in their attempts to think about sexual differences and the role of the biological or nature in the production of these.

As contemporary subjects of biopower, men and women in the West are increasingly subjectified through technoscientific and biomedical discourses around life. Like genes, although arguably less visibly, sex hormones play a significant role in these contemporary bio-subjectifications. Sex hormones, as this book will show, have been understood as one of the key actors in producing healthy, reproductive and sexually differentiated bodies since the early twentieth century. Indeed, hormonal systems are increasingly held to play key roles in bridging the gap between genes and bodies. Like genes, sex hormones also play a significant role in popular discourses around bodies. In everyday conversation and in cultural and media representations, sex hormones are understood as potent players in the production of human and non-human animal differences. They are thus key actors in the production of contemporary ways of being. The understanding of hormones as messengers of sex developed in this book provides a model for thinking the complex interrelations of the biological and the social that underpin such subjectifications, thus allowing for a more complex analysis of, and potential resistance towards, contemporary configurations of life.

PART I

Hormone histories

1

Folding hormonal histories of sex

The use of sex hormones to explain, refer to, or delimit sexual differences is, terminologically at least, specific to the twentieth century: the word 'hormone' was coined in Britain in 1905. The concept of chemical messengers of sex, however, is somewhat older than this. This chapter describes the development of this concept and shows how nineteenth- and early twentieth-century scientific theories about sex hormones were transmuted into strong claims about the determinative role of these chemicals in producing a broad range of physical, behavioural and psychological sexual differences in humans and other animals. This process involved the elision of more nuanced and less biologically determinist understandings of hormones as actors in producing sex. Through critically retelling a history of the hormonally sexed body, this chapter begins to investigate and elaborate both mainstream and alternative technoscientific figurations of hormones and to contribute to creating a 'history of bodies' in the Foucauldian sense, exploring what it might mean to think about bodies and 'the manner in which what is most material and most vital in them has been invested' (Foucault 1987: 152).

Histories of sexual differences

It has been claimed by historians of science, and most notably by Dutch science-studies theorist Nelly Oudshoorn (1994), that the 'discovery' or production of hormones in the early twentieth century marked a highly significant change in understandings of the nature of sexual difference. The naming of testosterone as the male sex hormone and oestrogen and progesterone as female sex hormones produced an understanding of masculinity and femininity as chemical. This was in stark contrast to older notions of sexual difference as being located throughout the body's organs, or more specifically in the reproductive organs. This change was part of a drastic rethinking of the nature of bodies and their production as differentiated. As British physiologist Ernest J. Starling (who coined the term hormone) wrote in 1923, it seemed

> almost a fairy tale that such widespread results, affecting every aspect of a man's life, should be conditioned by the presence or absence in the body of infinitesimal quantities of a substance which by its formula does not seem to stand out from the thousands of other substances with which organic chemistry has made us familiar.
>
> *(Starling, in Hall 1976: 277)*

Historically, it is useful to situate this change from a view of sexual difference as founded on sex organs or nerves to understandings of hormones as chemical messengers of sex within a better-known set of debates about physiological explanations of sexual difference. In *Making Sex: Body and Gender from the Greeks to Freud*, historian Thomas Laqueur (1992) argues that there was a shift in late eighteenth- and early nineteenth-century science and medicine from a one-sex model of sexual difference to a two-sex model. In the earlier model, which dates from the ancient Greeks, women were seen as equivalent to men except that, due to lack of heat, their (inferior) genitals were inside the body rather than outside. Women, in this model, were lesser versions of men. Historian Londa Schiebinger also describes this model, noting how examples of women who became men (when a penis suddenly came out of their body) were used to support this argument (Schiebinger 1989: 163–4).

The two-sex model, which originated in the mid to late eighteenth century, was quite different from this, as it posited a central and all-encompassing difference between the sexes – a difference needless to say that placed women, as if naturally, in an inferior position to men. Through the nineteenth century, in other words, the relation between the sexes moved from one of hierarchy to one of incommensurability and the notion of the sexes as 'opposite' was emphasised. The rise of this two-sex model was accompanied and in part produced by the detailed search for the biological proofs of indisputable difference. Schiebinger argues that in the late eighteenth century this search began with the investigation of the sexually differentiated nature of the skeleton (Schiebinger 1989: 191). In contrast to sixteenth-century drawings by Vesalius in which a human skeleton was used to represent males *and* females, anatomists of the eighteenth century drew skeletons that were sexually differentiated. Female skeletons were represented as having broader hips, narrower ribs and smaller skulls. Schiebinger suggests that this focus on the skeleton was part of a more general move away from the idea that sexual differences were only located in the sexual organs, towards their being located throughout the bones, flesh and organs. It was also strongly related to an emphasis on women's role in the domestic sphere: female skeletons were represented with hips suitable for childbearing, thus emphasising women's 'natural' proclivity for motherhood.

In her book *Sexual Science*, Cynthia Russett (1989) details the nineteenth-century versions of this two-sex model and the complex and diverse searches for definitive proof of the biological inferiority of women and non-European people.[1] Scientists spent much time in the nineteenth century looking at brain sizes, skeleton shape, energy levels, skull formation, performance on various physical and intellectual tests and the effects of menstruation and childbearing, amongst other things, to find the evidence they wanted. These scientists believed that sexual difference was everywhere in the body and could be located in various sites – not only in the obviously different reproductive systems, but in more obscure areas also.

Not coincidentally, the situation of women was also being widely debated at this time. Early European, North American and Australian feminists were arguing that women's unjustifiably poor social and political positions needed to change. There were differences of opinion amongst them, however, concerning the issue of sexual difference and much disagreement as to the cause of women's inferior position (Caine 1992; Bland 1995). Some feminists followed the two-sex model and agreed that women were fundamentally different from men, arguing that women thus had much that was unique to offer society. Others claimed that such differences were exaggerated and that equality in education and opportunity would prove that women were very similar to men. Anti-feminists, on the other hand, insisted that women's inferior social position was biologically decreed and so should remain unchanged. Medical and scientific evidence was cited by all sides, but it was the anti-feminist position that gained most support.[2] Mainstream doctors and scientists evinced a firm belief in the biological fixity of sexual difference and the 'naturalness' of corresponding

---

[1] Understandings of racial differences were entwined with these views of sexual difference in complex ways. This point is developed in Chapter 4 and in Roberts 2003a.

[2] Bland argues that late nineteenth- and early twentieth-century feminists only sometimes used medical statistics to support their arguments because they did not want to collude in women's reduction to their anatomy. Many feminists believed that only when there were more women doctors would the truth about the importance of the body in sexual difference be established (Bland 1995: 67–70).

social arrangements. These men intervened in social debates (for example, those around the education of women and the provision of birth control information) and issued pronouncements and treatments that accorded with the two-sex-model view.

The debates around the nature of sexual difference and the one-sex (or sameness) versus the two-sex (or radical difference) model were not restricted to the field of science. In the nineteenth century and into the turn of the twentieth century, these issues were central to feminism; indeed, as Donna Haraway writes, 'The history of modern feminism would be incomprehensible without the history of modern reproductive biology and clinical gynecology – as a moral discourse about social order and as a social technology' (Haraway 1989: 356–7). These debates were also linked to other forms of cultural politics such as the eugenics movement and early homosexual movements.

Internal secretions and internal environments

As well as searching for the bodily sites of racial and sexual differences, nineteenth-century physiologists and practitioners of the new science of biology were interested in the functioning of the body as a system. After discovering the glucose-producing function of the liver, French physiologist Claude Bernard in 1855 put forward the radical idea that the body produces chemicals that are needed for its own survival, and so is somewhat independent of its external environment (Canguilhem 1994: 85). He named these chemicals 'internal secretions'. Bernard argued that the body was an organism made up of disparate parts that functioned to keep its internal environment in a consistent state, 'compensating for deviations and perturbations' in order to remain in homeostasis (Canguilhem 1994: 85).

Philosopher of science Georges Canguilhem argues that the notions of the internal environment and homeostasis were central to the development of endocrinology. 'The concept that proved fruitful', he writes, 'was that of the internal environment, which, unlike the concept of internal secretion, was not closely associated with a specific function [such as the liver's production of glucose]; rather, from the first it was identified with another concept, that of a physiological constant' (Canguilhem 1994: 121). This notion of a stable internal environment led to 'the logical possibility . . . of transforming the concept of internal secretion into one of chemical regulation' (Canguilhem 1994: 121).

Although, as Canguilhem states, Bernard's theories created the 'logical possibility' of internal (chemical) secretions being responsible for bodily regulation (including, I would add, the regulation of sexual difference), the idea did not flourish until the turn of the century. Bernard did not see internal secretions as chemical regulators, but rather 'primarily as a reservoir of energy for the cells of the body' (Canguilhem 1988: 98). At this time, the nervous system was believed to regulate bodily functions and was held responsible for differences between men and women. Like other physiologists, Bernard believed that nerves (rather than chemicals) coordinated the organism. It was not until the 1890s that the notion of internal secretions was reinterpreted, sparking off the radical usurpation of the nervous system's role in the regulation of bodies and sexual difference.

Organotherapy

The 'founding story' of sex endocrinology is told by historian of endocrinology Victor Medvei thus: in June 1889, French physiologist Charles Brown- Séquard suggested to the Society of Biology in Paris that the testes contained an invigorating substance that could be removed from animals and injected into men as a rejuvenating agent (Medvei, 1982: 289).[3] Seventy-two-year-old Brown-Séquard had trialled this procedure on himself. 'Last first of June', he wrote, 'I sent to the Society of Biology a communication, which was followed by several others, showing the remarkable effects produced on myself by subcutaneous injection of a liquid obtained by the maceration on a mortar of the testicle of a dog or of a guinea pig to which one has added a little water' (in Medvei 1982: 289). The effects produced were improvements in strength, vigour and mental activity and increased contractibility of the bladder and intestine (Medvei 1982: 300). These experiments were part of an ongoing investigation into the effects of what came to be known as 'organotherapy', an important precursor of hormonal treatments.

Organotherapy, the practice of putting extracts from the organs of an animal into a human, was intended to remedy a supposed deficiency of the internal secretion produced by that organ. The therapy became a controversial and popular practice in the late nineteenth and early twentieth

---

[3] These ideas reflected both the commonly accepted notion that masturbation in men led to debility and loss of strength (Borell 1976: 235) and a long historical association of masculinity with the testes and their products (Oudshoorn 1994: 17–18). Oudshoorn points out that prior to the eighteenth century, treatments using testicular extracts were common and accepted, but 'by 1800, testicular extracts had disappeared from the official pharmacopoeias in Europe' (Oudshoorn 1994: 18). Potions made from these substances were still available from 'quacks', however, despite disapproval from the medical profession.

centuries.[4] In contrast to North America, the notion of organotherapy was not accepted in Britain until after the development of treatments for thyroid problems and diabetes using similar methods (Medvei 1982: 290–303).

According to historian of endocrinology Merriley Borell (1976), it was the developing field of physiology, trying to distinguish itself from clinical medicine, which took the notion of internal secretions into the laboratory at the end of the nineteenth century. The use of organ extracts to test notions of internal secretions established a new technology for the field. Initially, however, the notion that internal secretions played a role in sexuality and sexual differences was not accepted. English physiologist Edward Schaefer's experiments focused on the liver, kidney and pancreas as organs of internal secretion and he rejected Brown-Séquard's hypothesis regarding the sex glands. In an important speech to the British Medical Association in 1895 Schaefer did not mention the clinical studies done on the testicles or the ovaries and 'dismissed the idea that the sex glands produced internal secretions' (Borell 1976: 261). These glands, he and others still thought, caused their effects via the nervous system (Schaefer, in Medvei 1982: 335). Borell argues that this opinion was also influenced by what doctors and scientists perceived as the extravagant claims made in the popular press for organotherapy's rejuvenating effect on men (Borell 1985: 1–2, 8).[5]

This sequence of incidents shows that a scientific 'discovery' does not have an immediate or simple effect. Although Bernard first postulated the notion of internal secretions in 1855, it was not until 1889 that Brown-Séquard reported his experiments with dogs' testicles. In 1895 Schaefer

---

[4] Controversy centred not only around the scientific merit of these treatments, but also on moral questions concerning the use of animal extracts and the possibility that masturbation might be involved. There were also problems when Brown-Séquard claimed improvement in some nervous disorders, which fed concern that the effects were due to suggestion only (Borell 1985: 4). Borell notes that Brown-Séquard recommended sexual excitement without ejaculation to some of his patients. It seems there was concern then both about ejaculation, which caused loss of strength, and about sexual excitement without ejaculation (Borell 1976: 238–9). For a more detailed discussion of this concern with masturbation see Porter and Hall (1995: 132–77).

[5] The use of hormones to stimulate aging men's sexuality continued into the first decades of the twentieth century. In France and America, human, monkey and other animal testes were transplanted into men and animals in order to treat a wide range of ailments. Great controversy raged in the 1920s around a French practitioner, Serge Voronoff, who performed many of these operations (the so-called 'monkey gland affair'). This practice reportedly died out in the late 1930s (Hamilton 1986; Hoberman and Yesalis 1995: 62; Hirschbein 2000). This issue is taken up again in Part III.

was still assuming that sexuality and sexual difference were not controlled by internal secretions, but were matters of nerves. The progression from the notion of internal secretions to the 'discovery' of hormones themselves did not occur until after the turn of the century, despite it being 'a logical possibility' all that time. Borell puts this down to the expectation that the immediate cause of most responses of the body was a nervous stimulus: 'Until specific physiological responses were identified as needing explanation by other than nervous causation', she writes, 'physiologists *simply did not realize* that chemicals were capable of provoking physiological events in the same manner as nervous stimuli' (Borell 1985: 10, emphasis added). Although Borell's explanation seems weak ('not realizing' is rarely 'simple'), what is significant here is the fact that scientific thought around hormones did not proceed in a straightforward manner according to the availability of empirical data. The shift to a hormonal understanding of the body (and more specifically of sexual difference) was profound and one that was to encounter serious intellectual hurdles before becoming accepted as 'fact'.

Internal secretions and sex

In 1895, then, the theory that chemicals might control the body's functions remained highly controversial; internal secretions were not seen as regulators. In 1902, however, Schaefer's colleagues William Bayliss and Ernest Starling decided in studying the pancreas that chemicals could stimulate physiological events (Borell 1985: 10–11). They concluded that alongside the nervous system, there existed a system of chemical regulation operating via 'messengers' in the blood (Medvei 1982: 340). In 1905 Starling introduced the word 'hormone', based on the Greek *hormao*, meaning 'I excite or arouse' into physiological discourse. He defined hormones as chemical messengers carried in the bloodstream from the organ where they are produced to the organ where they have their effect. Hormones, he claimed, are produced and circulated by the body in order to satisfy recurring physiological needs (Borell 1985: 11). Two years later Schaefer accepted that it was 'highly probable that it is to internal secretions containing special hormones that the essential organs of reproduction – the testicles and the ovaries – owe the influence that they exert on the development of secondary sexual characters, and ... upon the maintenance in a well-developed condition of important internal organs of generation' (Schaefer, in Borell 1985: 13). In other words, he accepted that biological sexual difference was a matter of hormones, rather than nerves.

Borell argues that physiology had now claimed reproduction and, to some extent, sexuality, as legitimate parts of its field (Borell 1985: 16–17). By 1910 the move from internal secretions to hormones had been achieved. The definition of hormones as chemical messengers was taken up by physiologists who began the detailed work of 'discovering' individual hormones and establishing details regarding their production and effects. Borell writes, 'After 1910 no one seriously questioned the existence of testicular and ovarian hormones. However, selection of the strategy for discovery of each of these elusive substances was hotly debated' (Borell 1985: 18). Nelly Oudshoorn's book, *Beyond the Natural Body: An Archeology of Sex Hormones* (1994), documents this process.

'Discovering' sex hormones

Using social-network theory, Oudshoorn maps the influence of different scientific groups involved in early twentieth-century hormone research. Social-network theory suggests that rather than being 'discovered' in nature, scientific objects such as hormones are produced within networks of interactions amongst different groups. The process of writing scientific history involves mapping these social interactions. Oudshoorn also relies on the work of medical philosopher Ludwig Fleck to suggest that these interactions involve the incorporation of cultural ideas (what Fleck calls 'prescientific ideas'). Cultural beliefs about masculinity and femininity, for example, are taken on by scientists working on hormones, but are also actively transformed by scientific work (Oudshoorn 1994: 11–15).

Oudshoorn argues that gynaecologists were the first to work on the relevance of the theory of internal secretion to sex glands, especially in relation to women and ovarian secretions (Oudshoorn 1994: 19–20). Gynaecologists had long been interested in the role of the ovaries in sexuality and had observed changes that occurred after ovarectomy, a common medical practice in the late nineteenth century (Moscucci 1990: 134–64; Sengoopta 2000: 430). They also had a vested interest in learning about the ovarian secretions as such knowledge would give them greater control over their main object: women's reproductive systems. When physiologists took up the notion of sex hormones at the end of the first decade of the twentieth century, Oudshoorn argues, there was an important shift in the divisions between the two fields (gynaecology and physiology) that was to have a long-term effect on the medicalisation of women's bodies. This move, she suggests, meant that chemical treatments of women's bodies (specifically the use of hormones as medications) became cornerstones of gynaecological medicine. The entry of biochemists into the field of hormones was also important. In the 1920s, new biochemical techniques allowed for the extraction of steroid hormones from gonads (Hall 1976: 83). Significant also were networks formed with the pharmaceutical industry and gynaecological clinics for the provision of research materials to biochemistry laboratories (Oudshoorn 1994: 65–81). It was the networked combination of these four fields – gynaecology, physiology, biochemistry and pharmacy – that, Oudshoorn argues, produced hormones as we know them today.

The combined activities of these fields led to the chemical isolation of female sex steroids from the urine of horses and pregnant women in 1929 and to the isolation of male sex hormones from men's urine in 1931 (Oudshoorn 1994: 29). Initially, following the two-sex model, female sex hormones were thought to exist only in women (and indeed to cause femininity) and male sex hormones only in men. Sex chromosomes had been 'discovered' decades earlier, in 1902, by American zoologist Clarence I. McClung (Oudshoorn 1994: 156). According to historian Diana Long Hall, conflict occurred between geneticists and physiologists around the importance of chromosomes to sex determination. She claims it was the embryologists who provided the connections between the two groups, arguing that hormones could 'fill the gap' between genetics and sexed physiologies (Hall 1976: 85–6). In 1917 biologist Frank R. Lillie concluded that 'the "intentions" of the genes must always be carried through by appropriate hormones developed in the gonad' (Hall 1976: 87).

By the 1930s, then, sex hormones were seen 'as chemical messengers of masculinity and femininity' (Oudshoorn 1994: 22–3). Some endocrinologists went further, claiming that sex hormones had antagonistic effects on the bodies of 'the opposite sex'. Viennese physician Eugen Steinach, for example, performed experiments demonstrating that female hormones not only promoted female characteristics but also suppressed male ones (Steinach and Loebel 1940). Throughout the 1920s, however, there were increasing reports that this clear separation between the sexes did not exist: each sex was found to contain the 'other's' hormone (these were called 'heterosexual' hormones). In 1934 a report in *Nature* stated that the urine of stallions was a far better source of oestrogen than that of mares (Medvei 1982: 406). At the same time it was discovered that oestrogen and testosterone are chemically very similar and that testosterone is sometimes converted into oestrogen in the body. Although these findings resonated with contemporary understandings of sexual difference in sexology and psychoanalysis, they were reportedly received as 'startling' (Oudshoorn

1994: 26). The findings led to considerable confusion amongst scientists and doctors about the nature of sexual difference. (Male) homosexuality, for example, was used to explain the lack of clear hormonal division between the sexes. In the 1920s, biologists working in this area 'agreed ... that the sex hormones must be distinct and sex exclusive or their hosts would be abnormal: in the words of [biologist] Robert Frank, males whose blood passed the Allen/Doisy test [the test for blood-borne oestrogens] must be "latent homosexuals"' (Hall 1976: 89).

In 1939, however, a review of the current state of sex endocrinology stated:

> The present epoch has been characterized as one of confusion because of the demonstration of the close chemical interrelationships of all the sex hormones ... the possibility of the conversion of one to the other (it will be remembered that the urine of the stallion is one of the most potent sources of estrone, whereas it is not found in the urine of the gelding), the isolation of male hormone from actual ovarian tissue, and the fact that all males secrete estrogens and females androgens. All these matters are now well established facts.
>
> *(Herbert Evans, in Hall 1976: 91)*

It was now a 'well-established fact' that sexual differences were a matter of relative quantities of particular chemicals, rather than absolute essences. A model of a continuum between male and female along which individuals could be placed as more or less feminine or masculine had become dominant. This model led to the application of hormonal analysis to the study of the presumed femininity of homosexual men and (to a much lesser extent) the masculinity of lesbian women (Oudshoorn 1994: 56–9).[6] In the 1930s scientists also outlined the importance of the brain to hormonal systems and 'discovered' the gonadotropic hormones (those secreted by the pituitary gland), thus recognising the importance of the brain to the development of sexed bodies. For Oudshoorn, this conceptualisation of a feedback system between the brain and the gonads 'meant a definitive break with common-sense opinions that the essence of femininity and masculinity was located in the gonads' (Oudshoorn 1994: 37). Sexual difference was now seen to be located in chemicals rather than in organs or cells.

---

[6] This view of homosexuality was prevalent in sexology at this time. Hall and Porter argue that the move to viewing sexuality as a matter of chemicals made the study of sexuality more respectable, at least in Britain: sexuality 'could be presented as "scientifically interesting" without any necessary reference to the messy problems of human sexuality' (Hall and Porter 1995: 175). Hall and Porter see this as part of a general co-option of sexology into the less (outwardly) political field of scientific biology.

It might be thought that these established 'facts' would have meant the end of the two-sex model. The fact that we still refer to hormones as 'male' and 'female' today, however, shows a failure to shake off the notion of dualistic sexual difference that informed early endocrinology. The persistence of an 'old' notion of masculinity and femininity as dualistic is also evident in the fact that science still struggles to understand the role of 'heterosexual' hormones. How can this persistence be explained?

Understanding change: between 'science' and 'culture'

The move from a nineteenth-century notion of the neuronal body where dichotomous sexual difference is diffused throughout the body's organs, to a twentieth-century notion of a hormonal body where sexual difference is a matter of differential amounts of sex hormones, constitutes a significant change in understandings of human and other animal biology. In Foucault's terms, this change reconfigures the investment of materiality and vitality of bodies. But how we explain this reconfiguration?

Conventional histories of endocrinology describe this change but do not adequately explain it. As quoted earlier, Borell writes that, prior to 1902, physiologists 'simply did not realize' that chemicals could act as messengers in the body (Borell 1985: 10), which does not constitute a substantive explanation. Medvei (1982), in a conventional historiographic way, posits the change as a matter of internal scientific progress and individual achievement. His explanation does not give us any sense of the ways in which changes within endocrinology relate to any other factors. The standard alternative to this conventional approach is to examine the social context of the scientific developments. It might be possible, for example, to read nineteenth-century science's positing of an innate and unchangeable difference between men and women as a political act to justify women's limited social positions in the face of feminist agitation. One could then read the change over the turn of the century as reflective of an acknowledgement of the similarities between men and women, as women proved that they were capable of intellectual and other achievements of standards equivalent to those of men.[7]

---

[7] Russett describes how in the early twentieth century, feminist psychologists (men and women) demonstrated that women could perform equally to men on intellectual and other tests. The women's own records of achievements at universities also helped to prove this point (Russett 1989).

This style of explanation is common in feminist histories of science. In *The Mind Has No Sex*, for example, Schiebinger writes '[M]y hope is that this book will ... shed light on how gender relations have molded (and continue) to mold scholarship and knowledge more generally. The nature of science is no more fixed than the social relations of men or women: science too is shaped by social forces' (Schiebinger 1989: 9).[8] Russett also positions science as a tool used by culture to explain cultural differences between men and women (Russett 1989: 10). Although advocating a more interactive model between ideas and social change elsewhere in the book (Russett 1989: 179), Russett's concluding sentences are telling: 'The construction of womanhood by Victorian scientists grew out of and was responsive to the very human needs of a particular historical moment. It needs to be seen for the masculine power play that it was, but it needs to be seen also as an intellectual monument, etched in fear, of the painful transition to the modern world view' (Russett 1989: 206).[9] Here, Russett uses 'culture' to explain scientific thought.

The science studies approach: Latour, Oudshoorn and Haraway

These feminist histories of science split culture and science and posit science as an effect of culture. This approach creates a circularity in which science is explained by cultural anxieties, the evidence of which is the content of science. The problem this split poses for any analysis of

---

[8] Schiebinger makes a similar argument in the introduction to her subsequent book *Nature's Body* (Schiebinger 1993: 1–10).

[9] This approach to scientific history is often influenced (sometimes without explicit discussion) by psychoanalytic thinking. This is evident in the loose but persistent use of terms such as 'anxiety' and 'projection'. In discussing the American Medical Association's view of abortion in 1860–80, for example, Carroll Smith-Rosenberg writes, 'The A.M.A. scripted social anxieties onto the physical and into the text. But the historian must ask, which anxieties?' The AMA's views on abortion are theorised as an anxious response to threat of the 'New Woman'. Smith-Rosenberg uses terms directly from psychoanalysis – 'Having *projected* the problematic aspects of the bourgeois revolution ... onto the mystified figure of the aborting matron'; 'The True Woman counterpoised a mystified past to an *anxious* present in a sexual rhetoric that bespoke the discursive *compulsions* and ideological *conflicts* of an actual past' (Smith-Rosenberg 1989: 105–6, emphases added) – without any discussion of how such an enormous move between the subject and culture can be understood. Out of this lack of discussion another problem arises: oppositional discourses are seen to be more rational or 'truthful' than the anxious or compulsive moves of scientists or doctors. Thus Smith-Rosenberg describes the views of nineteenth-century women as 'Expressing what may well have been the *actual* sexual concerns of many of their readers' (Smith-Rosenberg 1989: 107) and suggests that although these women also constructed discourses around sexuality, theirs had a more rational connection to the truth of women's lives than did the discourses of doctors.

science has become an important focus for science studies over the past two decades. French sociologist of science and technology, Bruno Latour, is a major figure in this debate.

Latour's main criticism of the 'cultural context of science' approach is that to discuss only the context of science 'would once again be to filter the content of a science, keeping only its social environment' (Latour 1988: 8). Against this, his historical method attempts to avoid the content/context distinction, arguing that the notion that the two are separate is a historically produced idea. Although this notion marks the birth of modernity, the fact that the distinction can never be maintained, Latour suggests, shows that 'we have never been modern' (the title of his 1993 book). Culture has just as much of a history and is as much socially constructed as science and therefore cannot be used as an explanation of what happens in science (see also Latour 1990).

That context cannot be used as an explanation for science does not mean that science is separate from culture, but rather that it is always involved in the production of culture. In writing about physics, Latour states that 'If there is one thing the particle physicists do not do it is *reflect* their existing culture; this does not mean that they escape the confines of the collective, but that they are building a *different* collective' (Latour 1990: 168). This is why the sciences exclude social analysis – they 'revolutionize the very concept of society and of what it comprizes' (Latour 1988: 38). In the work of producing 'the microbe' for example, '[I]n the great upheaval of late nineteenth-century Europe … [scientists] redefine what society is made up of, who acts and how, and they become the spokesmen for these new innumerable, invisible, and dangerous agents' (Latour 1988: 39; see also Latour 1983: 159–69).

As an alternative to the analysis of the cultural context of science, Latourian actor-network theory posits all entities and enterprises as part of a network of forces in which no part has ontological primacy. Thus scientists, farmers and hygiene activists are all indispensable to the production of a scientific artefact such as the 'microbe'. Latour refuses also to make a distinction between human and non-human in his examination of scientific history. For him they are all 'actors' and 'allies'.[10] For example, in his history of Pasteur, Latour (1988) includes as allies of the scientists and as actors in the story of the 'discovery' of 'microbes', hygienists,

---

[10] This inclusion of non-human entities as actors distinguishes the actor-network theory approach from the social network approach employed by Oudshoorn, whose analysis is restricted to interactions between human actors (Oudshoorn 1994: 153–4).

drains, Agar gels, chickens, farms and insects. All of these, he says, were integral to the production of the microbe as a scientific object (Latour 1988: 147).

Applying actor-network theory to the history of science involves examining the interplay and interdependencies of these actors and allies. Latour looks at how the different social groups (scientists, doctors, farmers) 'translate' ideas or actors to suit their own needs. These interactions are all about forces and about usefulness: if a new actor (for example, the microbe) can be used to achieve things in a faster way, it will be taken on board. And this is also true for the actors themselves. If the microbe is put into Agar gel in the laboratory, its interests are served and it will grow. Latour argues that each social group has its own interpretation of the actor, but that such translations are necessary to the survival of a scientific 'discovery'. Such 'discoveries' need to be connected to other things, to be moved by other forces, to become valid and to have an effect: The actor 'requires a force to fetch it, seize upon it for its own motives, move it, and often transform it' (Latour 1988: 16). Latour's most famous metaphor for this process is that of a train track. 'Scientific facts are like trains', he argues, 'they do not work off their rails. You can extend the rails and connect them but you cannot drive a locomotive through a field' (Latour 1983: 155).

Latour also argues that a new actor will not be taken on until it can do everything and explain everything that the old actor could do and explain. The 'discovery' of a new actor then (such as the microbe) requires that older ideas and practices (such as those around miasmas as causes of illness) are *replaced*. Latour writes, 'To discover the microbe is not a matter of revealing at last the "true agent" *under* all the other, now "false" ones. In order to discover the "true" agent, it is necessary in addition to show that the new translation also includes all the manifestations of the earlier agents and to put an end to the argument of those who want to find it other names' (Latour 1988: 81, emphasis in original). In other words, 'To discover is not to lift the veil. It is to construct, to relate, and then to "place under"' (1988: 81).

These ideas provide new purchase on the difficult shift within scientific discourse from theories of internal secretions to understanding hormones as messengers. As described above, Bernard's 1855 'discovery' of internal secretions was not taken up until the early twentieth century. At this time there were numerous social groups ready to translate the actor of internal secretions to suit their own needs. As Oudshoorn (1994) documents, in the early twentieth century the discipline of physiology was more firmly established, gynaecological clinics existed and were willing to provide women's urine for laboratories to study and the pharmaceutical industry had begun to recognise the market potential for hormonal treatments.[11] Similarly, as is described in Chapter 6, sexologists and theorists of homosexuality were producing a notion of the 'third sex' that fitted in well with endocrinological research in which homosexuals were described as belonging to a hormonal 'third sex' lying between male and female. The successful 'discovery' of hormones was made possible by the willingness of these groups to take on and translate this actor.

Latour argues that although these other social allies are necessary to the development of a scientific idea, they are usually then left outside the official histories of the science: 'These allies, of which the science is sometimes ashamed, are almost always outside the magic circle by which it later, after its victory, redefines itself' (Latour 1988: 59–60).[12] Thus official histories of endocrinology do not describe the inputs of gynaecological clinics or the abattoirs that supplied animal gonads. They do not emphasise the perceived needs of patients as important to the development of laboratory research. In this, science manages to appear to be separate from culture and to feed ideas or 'discoveries' back to culture. In contradiction to this tradition, Latour writes in relation to Pasteur's work on the microbe that 'Pasteur's work does not "emerge in society" to "influence" it. It was already in society; it never ceases to be so' (Latour 1988: 91).

Latour's thinking about the problems of a culture/science split is convincing and his comments regarding a social context approach to scientific history are important. Donna Haraway, however, has some reservations about Latour's approach. She argues that in his desire to avoid describing (or producing) the social context of science, Latour ends up giving an unbalanced emphasis to the technical side of science. This means that many political questions are left untouched. In a footnote to her article, 'The Promises of Monsters', she writes:

> Correctly working to resist a 'social' explanation of 'technical' practice by exploding the binary, these scholars [Latour and other major figures in science

---

[11] This is discussed in detail in relation to the development of hormone-replacement therapies in Chapter 4.

[12] This strategy is also used by scientists at the time. Latour argues, for example, that despite making alliances with hygienists, government and farmers and relying on these alliances and their translations of his work, Pasteur always claimed that everything he did came only from science. 'This double strategy bears the stamp of genius', Latour writes, 'for it amounts to translating the wishes of practically all the social groups of the period, then getting those wishes to emanate from a body of pure research that did not even know it was applicable to or comprehensible by the very groups from which it came' (Latour 1988: 71).

studies] have a tendency covertly to reintroduce the binary by worshipping only one term – the 'technical'. Especially, *any* consideration of matters like masculine supremacy or racism or imperialism or class structures are inadmissible because they are the old 'social' ghosts that blocked real explanation of science in action . . . I agree with Latour and [Michael] Lynch that practice creates its own context, but they draw a suspicious line around what gets to count as 'practice'. They *never* ask how the *practices* of masculine supremacy, or many other systems of structured inequality, get *built* into and out of working machines . . . Systems of exploitation might be crucial parts of the 'technical content' of science.

(Haraway 1992a: 332, emphasis in original)[13]

This pertinent criticism could also be applied to Oudshoorn's history of sex hormones. Whilst Oudshoorn's social network analysis tells a new story of hormones that successfully indicates that these were not 'discovered' in nature, but rather were produced through scientific interaction and work, the line she draws around networks of practice tends to leave important questions open. In relation to the point that significantly more work was undertaken around female hormones than male hormones, for example, Oudshoorn argues that this was due to the ability of scientists, gynaecologists and pharmaceutical companies to set up functioning networks around women's bodies. The fact that gynaecological clinics could easily collect the urine of pregnant women meant that biochemists could be supplied with materials to work with. Male urine, on the other hand, was difficult to collect, as there were no equivalent institutions focussing on male bodies. Thus Oudshoorn makes a highly practical point: concentration of work on female hormones was due to the availability of networks that could supply research materials. Without denying the importance of such practical matters, this argument begs a key question: why were clinics set up around women's bodies and not around men's? Which '*practices* of masculine supremacy, or . . . other systems of structured inequality' were built into this practical fact?[14]

---

[13] More recently, Haraway notes that this overdue attention to feminist thinking is beginning to take place in science studies: 'In particular, in writing and speaking in the mid-1990s, Latour, as well as . . . several other scholars, evidence serious, nondefensive interest in feminist science studies, including the criticism of their own rhetorical and research strategies in the 1980s' (Haraway 1997: 279). In my experience of the field of STS in Europe, the United States and Australia over the last decade, there is still far to go in terms of recognition of feminist arguments in much STS research.

[14] In various places in *Beyond the Natural Body*, Oudshoorn also reverts to descriptions that separate 'culture' and 'science' (see, for example, Oudshoorn 1994: 114–15). Although scientists take on prescientific (cultural) ideas, they 'thoroughly transform' these (Oudshoorn 1994: 34) and then feed these new ideas back to society. This temporal

One way to answer such questions is to emphasise the significance of the embodied location of the scientist: in Haraway's terms to understand technoscience as 'situated knowledge' (Haraway 1991). This approach posits scientific and other knowledges as always embodied and therefore coming from a specific, marked position. Haraway uses the metaphor of vision, arguing that the embodied vision of scientific practices is not a 'natural' or innocent one, but is active and selective. In later work, she contrasts this situated non-innocent point of view with the modern understanding of the scientist as a 'modest witness', described by Steven Shapin and Simon Schaffer in their book *Leviathan and the Air-Pump* (1985). Shapin and Schaffer argue that mainstream understandings of the objective scientist were developed by Robert Boyle in seventeenth-century England. The scientist is described as a modest witness because he is able to approach the world in an entirely objective, non-emotional manner. Discussing Elizabeth Potter's history of the same period, Haraway (1997) argues that Shapin and Schaffer fail to understand the ways in which this version of the scientist as a modest witness is implicated in the production of gendered, raced and classed forms of embodiment. Boyle's objective observer is necessarily a white, middle-class male.

In naming her book *Modest_Witness@Second_Millennium*, Haraway reappropriates and reconfigures this term. 'I would like to queer the elaborately constructed and defended confidence of this civic man of reason', she writes, 'in order to enable a more corporeal, inflected, and optically dense, if less elegant, kind of modest witness to matters of fact to emerge in the worlds of technoscience' (Haraway 1997: 24). Reappropriating the modest witness and insisting that the reproduction of gender, race and class implicit in his origins are acknowledged, Haraway moves the scientist forward into the twenty-first century. Acknowledging his/her embodied location and, more importantly, paying attention to the ways in which what he/she *does* (re)produces certain versions of sex, race and class, means that the scientist can become a modest witness in a more politically engaged sense.

The figuration of the scientist as a modest witness and scientific knowledge as situated allows for an understanding of how science is involved with, or replicates, social dominations. A focus on embodied location helps to explain, for example, the persistence in scientific theories of sexual difference of certain ideas about the feminine or women, throughout

distinction implies an allegiance to a more fundamental split. The exclusion of non-human actors, such as hormones, facilitates this tendency through maintaining a space where practical activities surrounding and producing hormones are scientific or technical, rather than cultural.

centuries of different scientific actors. Although network theories can map
the movements and interactions that produce particular scientific artefacts, the persistence of notions across epochs seems difficult to explain
within these approaches. Indeed, such persistence may require a different
notion of time and history than that implied in actor or social network
approaches.

Time and embodiment in hormone histories

> The point is to learn to remember that we might have been otherwise, and might
> yet be, as a matter of embodied fact.
>
> *(Haraway 1997: 39)*

In a series of interviews with Latour, French philosopher of science Michel
Serres discusses his theory of time as 'folded, wadded up' (Serres, with
Latour 1995: 63). This theory stands in contradiction to a classical notion
that relates time to geometry, understanding time as a linear progression.
As an alternative, Serres thinks of time in a topological fashion, with rifts,
mountains and valleys. He uses a handkerchief as a model:

> If you take a handkerchief and spread it out in order to iron it, you can see in it
> certain fixed distances and proximities. If you sketch a circle in one area, you
> can mark out nearby points and measure far-off distances. Then take the same
> handkerchief and crumple it, by putting it in your pocket. Two distant points
> suddenly are close, even superimposed. If, further, you tear it in certain places,
> two points that were close can become very distant. This science of nearness and
> rifts is called topology, while the science of stable and well-defined distances is
> called metrical geometry.
>
> *(Serres 1995: 60)*

Serres' contention is that time is more like the crumpled handkerchief than
the ironed one and his readings of scientific history are based on this
understanding. Rather than assume that science proceeds in a linear fashion where the distances between events are even and constant, he suggests
that sciences always combine aspects that are archaic and before their time –
that the spaces between past, present and future are crumpled, or folded.
As a simple example, he takes the car, usually a symbol of up-to-the-minute
modernity and argues:

> It is a disparate aggregate of scientific and technical solutions dating from
> different periods. One can date it component by component: this part was
> invented at the turn of the century, another, ten years ago, and Carnot's cycle is
> almost two hundred years old. Not to mention that the wheel dates back to

neolithic times. The ensemble is only contemporary by assemblage, by its
design, its finish, sometimes only by the slickness of the advertising
surrounding it.

(Serres 1995: 45)

Historical eras, he says, are like the car: 'multitemporal, simultaneously
drawing from the obsolete, the contemporary, and the futuristic', revealing
'a time that is gathered together, with multiple pleats' (Serres 1995: 60).

This understanding transforms my retelling of the history of hormonal
explanations of sexual difference in two significant ways. Firstly, using the
notion of folded time, it becomes possible to argue that the history of a
science is *not* replaced as the science progresses through various translations (as Latour might be read to suggest), but rather is carried through
in at least some of its aspects, retaining a power beyond that to which
scientists and historians of science might admit. This means that time lags
in moving from theories of internal secretions to understanding hormones
as messengers of sex need be considered neither as unusual nor as a matter
of scientists 'simply not realizing' something significant, as Borell suggested. If time is folded and materialised as such within objects (like cars,
or in the hormone case, oestrogen or testosterone), then it makes perfect
sense that scientists continued to think about nerves and internal secretions despite mounting evidence about hormones that later indicated their
unique function as messengers of sex.

Secondly, the idea of folded time illuminates the lingering of notions of
dichotomous sexual difference in twentieth-century endocrinology,
despite the changes in understandings of hormonal physiology undermining this view. This lingering is due to the fact that other networks of
cultural meanings around sexual difference (including political, literary,
social scientific and religious discourses and practices) connect into and
affect the networks of scientific interactions that Oudshoorn describes so
well. Accepting this means that Oudshoorn's argument regarding the
existence of gynaecological clinics for women (and the absence of equivalent clinics for men) and the practical importance this had for endocrinology takes on a different light. This fact has significance not only in a
practical sense, but also insofar as it reveals some shared assumptions
about women's bodies, health and the role of science and medicine in
dealing with 'women's problems' that are deeply interwoven with endocrinological understandings of sexed bodies. As is argued in Part III of this
book, conceptions of particular hormonal processes shared by many women
as inherently pathological have underpinned vast networks of drug manu-
facture, medical treatment and personal experiences of reproduction and

aging for millions of women in the mid- to late-twentieth century. To understand the persistence of 'old' ideas about the sexes as opposite and complementary in the face of such significant transformation in scientific understandings of bodies, in other words, we need to look beyond the specific networks involved in the production of hormones and investigate the ways in which these are cross-cut by other networks of meaning-production and material work. As many historians of sex/gender have demonstrated, these networks – including those of sexology, psychoanalysis, feminism, religion, literature and politics – do not share a progressive narrative in relation to conceptualising sexual difference; rather, discourses of sexual difference have always been mixed up, contradictory, incoherent – in Serres' terms, crumpled or folded. Contemporary discourses and practices of hormonal bodies, I will argue, still bear the traces of these folded inconsistencies.

This suggestion that understanding the history of scientific actors such as sex hormones requires acknowledgement of the other scientific and non-scientific networks linking to the networks working directly on, and constituted by, the actor itself, begs the question as to how such networks make material differences to the central players. Conceptualising science as situated knowledge is powerful here, as the persistence of the two-sex model in endocrinology demonstrates. Haraway's theorisation of the embodied nature of scientific knowledge allows for the persistence of old ideas (or in Serres' terms, the crumpling of time) through recognising the embodiment of the scientist and all other actors and social groups. The term 'embodiment' does not refer here to a biological or psychological condition. It attempts to avoid this distinction, referring more to what Moira Gatens, following sociologist Pierre Bourdieu, describes as habitus, an unconscious accretion of cultural habits (Gatens 1996: x–xii), or to what Butler (1993) calls iterative, performative acts. As these philosophers show, embodiment is historical in a way that goes beyond personal life experience or individual or family psychology. Thus accounting for embodiment does not mean that personal details regarding the scientist should be given great weight – network theorists rightly reject the traditional emphasis on personal details in scientific history (Latour 1983: 157) – but rather that it matters how scientists are in play as located and embodied actors. 'Situatedness does not mean parochialism or localism', Haraway clarifies, 'but it does mean specificity and consequential, if variously mobile, embodiment' (Haraway 1997: 199). In Gatens' terms, for example (which, although not specifically used by Haraway, illuminate her argument here), the embodiment of any individual is a conglomeration of habits that take place in a particular historical location and that contain memories or folds of other historical times within them. Taking into account the scientist's embodiment, then, we can see that s/he is never only positioned in one network (that relating to the scientific discovery in question) but is also within many others simultaneously. Networks of scientific 'discovery' are not flat and linear, like Latour's train-track metaphor, but are more like Serres' three-dimensional crumpled handkerchief, with networks of connections running over and through them.

This view allows for a more satisfying history of sex hormones. Both network theory and the concept of folded time allow us to make more sense of the time delays between Bernard's 'discovery' of internal secretions, Brown-Séquard's self-injections and the acceptance of the notion of sex hormones as 'messengers of sex'. Network theories are important in their emphasis on networks of actors that must take up any scientific idea, whilst Serres' notion of folded time allows histories to move away from an expectation of sequential development. An emphasis on embodiment, however, provides another cornerstone to the history of bodies and specifically how, to re-cite Foucault, their materiality and vitality became invested through hormones. Contemporaneous understandings of sexual and other differences coming from sexology, feminism, eugenics and psychoanalysis are ignored in most histories of endocrinology. A view of science as embodied knowledge makes possible the argument that these disciplines and the actors moving within and across them had a significant impact on the development of endocrinological theories and practices and thus that networks outside those immediately connected with endocrinology are important to the history of the hormonal body. This kind of argument is elaborated in Part III of this book in relation to hormone-replacement therapies and environmental oestrogens.

The model of science as embodied knowledge allows for an understanding of the implication of science in social dominations and thus also for the possibility of rewritings. As Haraway writes, situatedness or location is about being 'partial in the sense of being *for* some worlds and not others' (Haraway 1997: 37). Although location is never self-evident or simple, it is finite and does provide the possibility of particular views. Serres' theory of time adds a further dimension to this argument – one that allows us to see how scientific history remains central to contemporary science. Situated knowledges, then, must also be genealogical ones in a Foucauldian sense: we need to know the history of hormones in order to see how this history is folded into present endocrinological and biomedical science.

Knowing the history of the networks around endocrinology is vital to understanding contemporary technoscientific and biomedical discourses and to producing ways of 'being otherwise'. The history of biological bodies is important precisely because it shows – in contradistinction to the ideas of the historians with which I began this chapter – the *lack* of separation between scientific representations and the materiality of bodies. In tune with Foucault's suggestions about body histories, my analysis of the history of the hormonally sexed body demonstrates *not* that science reflects culture through representation, but that material and vital bodies are produced through networks that fold and cut across technoscientific, biomedical and other fields. Hormonal sexual difference is always, to use Haraway's phrase, an 'embodied fact' produced within these intersecting networks (Haraway 1997: 39).

The narratives told in this chapter describe the historical production of the hormonally sexed body and these narratives are taken up again in Part III. Part II takes a closer look at how the hormonally sexed body is understood within technoscience and biomedicine today, discussing con-temporary explanations of hormones' involvement in messaging sex in human and non-human animal bodies and elaborating how hormones are figured as key in the production of sexual differences in foetuses, children and adults. In this Part I discuss what became of the early twentieth-century determinist view of hormones, exploring its instantia-tion as a full-blown set of technoscientific and biomedical discourses in the late twentieth century. I suggest that the more radical possibilities of understanding hormones as messengers within bio-social (rather than simply biological) systems are continually elided in mainstream techno-science and biomedical discourses, despite being, to borrow Canguilhem's phrase, 'a logical possibility' all the time. Engaging with this sense of possibility begins to put flesh on a reconfigured conception of hormones as (active) messengers of sex.

PART II

Hormonal bodies

Hormonal bodies

2

Articulating endocrinology's body

Stories and facts do not naturally keep a respectable distance; indeed, they promiscuously cohabit the same very material places. Determining what constitutes each dimension takes boundary-making and maintenance work. In addition, many empirical studies of technoscience have disabled the notion that the word *technical* designates a clean and orderly practical or epistemological space. Nothing so productive could be so simple.

(Haraway 1997: 68)

Across the twentieth century, hormones came to be seen as messengers of sex. As such, they figure today as key players in maintaining the biological life of human and non-human animals. Sex hormones are understood as essential both to the development and maintenance of healthy foetal, child and adult bodies and to the very possibility of sexual reproduction. This chapter examines contemporary technoscientific representations of the messaging actions of sex hormones. Working with contemporary theories of scientific knowledge production, it suggests that explanations of hormonal messaging contain unrealised potentialities for recognising the significant interweaving of 'the social' and 'the biological' constituting this messaging. In focusing attention on the intricate and microscopic patterns of hormonal flows, biologists and physiologists attempt to leave the social aside – to create, as Haraway puts it, 'respectable distance' between these explanatory categories. Close examination, however, shows that this 'clean ... epistemological space' is never fully achieved. Indeed, 'nothing so productive could be so simple': biological explanations of hormonal actions are always articulated with the social, both in their epistemologies and in their production as technoscientific knowledge.

Theorising technoscientific knowledge production

Modern western science attempts to represent nature or the world objectively. This goal is supported by a dualist philosophy that describes a distinction between body and mind and assumes that knowing can therefore be separated from the bodily experience of the knower. The scientific method is aimed at reduction of all biases and claims are made that if this method is accurately followed, the knowledge produced will not bear the marks of its producer. This notion is tied to an understanding of progress in which scientific knowledge is held to be gradually improving through the application of rational approaches to experimentation and theory building. Thus the historical position of the scientist is not considered relevant to science, except insofar as the 'mistakes' of the past can be put down to incorrect applications of the scientific method, or to the lack of technological knowledge and apparatuses. This view also assumes and reproduces a binary distinction between activity and passivity: the active (yet neutral) scientist represents the passive world or nature.

This view of scientific objectivity has been strongly criticised by philosophers and social scientists and in particular by feminists. In an extension of feminist standpoint theory, for example, philosopher Sandra Harding criticises the notion that who the scientist is has no impact on the science he or she produces (Harding 1986, 1991, 1993a). Standpoint theory argues that all knowledge is produced from a particular position from which certain values are more or less obvious. This position is not a personal one necessarily, but may be produced by a community (of American biologists, for example). Harding argues that because of this, science must view the *subjects* of science with as much critical interest as it does its objects. Harding's position does not view the politics of scientific knowledge brought about by different standpoints negatively (as do some other feminist approaches), but rather sees them as positive insofar as they can be changed, that is, insofar as the standpoints of marginalised groups can be substituted for those of dominant ones. The question 'Who is this knowledge for?' carries as much weight as 'What is the knowledge?' This is not, however, an endorsement of relativism – Harding instead argues that knowledges have different values and effects and that these should be examined in the analysis of science.[1]

---

[1] Harding's continued use of the word 'objectivity' in her description of what science from marginalised standpoints can produce is somewhat confusing in that it seems to imply a belief in objective rather than subjective views of the world or nature. However, Harding's position arguably has nothing to do with this dichotomy in its traditional mode (Bhavnani and

Haraway agrees that science is not neutral; her contention, based on empirical studies of the production of scientific knowledge, is that achieving modern forms of scientific objectivity 'takes boundary-making and maintenance work' (Haraway 1997: 68). Such studies demonstrate the fundamental point that science is produced through the interactions of embodied persons with things, texts and animals, all of which are materially and discursively situated within particular times and places. Accordingly, Haraway suggests that scientists rethink and rename what they do when they work with objects, animals or environments (or 'nature'). Rather than attempting to *represent* nature in a neutral way, scientists could understand their work as producing *articulations with* nature. This suggestion breaks down the traditional view of nature as passive and of 'all agency [being] ... firmly on the side of humanity' (Haraway 1992a: 304) and instead posits the world or nature as an active (although unlike) partner who 'is crucial to the generativity of the collective' that is science (Haraway 1992a: 313).

This chapter analyses contemporary technoscientific figurations of the activities of hormones in producing sexual differences. Developing Haraway's notion of technoscience as articulation, I discuss how these activities could be rethought, attributing a broader, more bio-social understanding of hormones' messaging actions. In so doing, the chapter investigates and begins to deconstruct two binary distinctions central to contemporary mainstream science: that between 'stories and facts' and that between the biological and the social. The analysis of contemporary scientific writing shows that technoscientific understandings of the role of hormones in human and non-human bodies are indeed complex and not, as some social scientific and feminist writing assumes, purely 'biological'. It shows, in other words, that technoscientific understandings of hormonal systems rely at least to some extent on the social as well as the biological. This is true not only in the sense that all discourse is cultural, but also that

Haraway 1994). This is particularly apparent in Harding's description of the object of science as 'nature as an object of knowledge' (Harding 1993a: 64) and in her insistence on the contradictory multiplicity and heterogeneity of the subjects of science and on their historically located embodiment. These understandings indicate that Harding's 'objectivity' is a long way from any traditional notions of neutrality and subjectivity. In the conclusion to her article, Harding argues that her use of the word 'objectivity' is intended to emphasise the repressed non-dominant political and intellectual history of this word. In this understanding objectivity does not relate to an absolute split between subject and object, but rather tries to keep open the gap between the knower and the world: 'The notion of objectivity is useful in providing a way to think about the gap that should exist between how any individual or group wants the world to be and how it in fact is' (Harding 1993a: 74).

there is space within endocrinological explanations for the intervention of the social into the production of sexed bodies (although this space is constantly underplayed or belied in technoscientific texts). Following Haraway and Harding, I read these technoscientific knowledges as cultural and as articulations coming from particular standpoints that produce particular embodiments, of both human and non-human entities. Endocrinology's hormonal body is produced culturally, although not only by human domination (representation) but also through the action of hormones themselves. The articulations that presently exist between nature and science regarding hormones and sexual differences are limited and limiting, but in their very situatedness, their standpoints, they are inherently moveable. In re-reading this story, we can begin to see possibilities for different articulations.

Contemporary physiology's hormonal body

How do the technoscientific fields of physiology and endocrinology describe the hormonal body? How do these fields answer the key questions: What is a hormone? How do hormones constitute or affect the body? And how are they related to sexual differences?

This chapter relies principally on various editions of two popular undergraduate physiology textbooks (Sherwood 1989, 1997, 2007; Van de Graaf and Fox 1989). It also refers to recent research papers in endocrinology and critical analyses of this literature. Whilst scientific fields cannot be reduced to the simplified and pedagogical content of textbooks, these provide important entries into understanding the basic principles and 'mindsets' of technoscientific fields. As science-studies theorist Bonnie B. Spanier writes:

> Biology textbooks construct mindsets for the next generation of scientists, physicians, and dentists. These books define the 'important' questions, the framework within which these questions are addressed, and the specific knowledge required to be a functioning scientist in the field. The values and ideologies embedded in textbooks may be responsible for alienating students who, for various reasons, do not resonate to these implicit and explicit assumptions. In this way, textbooks can act as a selective filter for serious science initiates, encouraging and inspiring some while discouraging others.
> *(Spanier 1995: 37)*

Textbook representations of hormones' role in producing biological differences are fundamental to endocrinology and physiology, developing an assumed knowledge base for more detailed research papers. Critically reading undergraduate textbooks provides access to the basic accepted 'stories and facts' of the relevant scientific fields.

What are hormones and how do they affect the body?

Moving from feminist critiques of technoscience to textbooks of physiology is a strange journey. It is a journey from professed uncertainty and wide-ranging ideas and examples, to a clear and narrowly focused set of principles and accepted truths. Suddenly, text is clarified by drawings and diagrams and readers are offered summaries and revision questions and colour-coded keywords. These are facts to be memorised and reproduced in the elsewhere of the examination room and medical or scientific life. It is difficult, to say the least, not to be seduced by the level of certainty and clarity that is offered in these descriptions of biological systems.

This section investigates the limits of this certainty and demonstrates that within these understandings of the endocrine system there are important areas of uncertainty that are belied by the textbooks' pedagogical tone. Even within textbook descriptions of basic biological processes, there is space for the intermixing of the social with the biological (specifically here in the unknown roles of neural and hormonal inputs to the brain's neurohormonal control system). This space problematises the scientific attempt to designate the 'orderly epistemological space' of a purely biological (i.e. non-social) description of human biology, and to provide descriptions that can separate stories and facts.

Within introductory physiology textbooks, hormones are defined as biologically active chemicals that are secreted into the blood by endocrine glands in response to an appropriate signal. They are carried in the blood to another set of cells (the target tissue or cells) where they affect the metabolism of these cells and thus modify the production or action of specific products (enzymes and other proteins) of these target cells. This movement is usually represented by arrows in line diagrams or flow charts (Sherwood 2007: 660, 760).[2] Hormones are divided into three groups, according to what they are made of: (1) amines – derivatives of the amino acid tryosine (an example is thyroid gland hormones); (2) polypeptides and glycoproteins – made from chains of specific amino acids of varying length (an example is insulin); and (3) steroids – made of neutral lipids derived from cholesterol (examples are the sex steroids testosterone and oestrogen).

---

[2] To see other examples, type 'endocrine system image' into an internet search engine.

What hormones are made of determines how they function in the body. The largest group – the polypeptides and glycoproteins – are water-soluble (hydrophilic), which means that they can be dissolved in the aqueous portion of the plasma in the blood and thus travel easily through the body. The steroids, on the other hand, are hydrophobic. They are lipids and cannot dissolve in the blood. They have to be attached to plasma-carrier proteins that carry them through the blood. This difference in constitution also affects the hormones' actions when they arrive at the target cell. Steroids, being lipids, can easily move through the target cell membrane, which is also partially lipid.

The glands from which hormones are secreted are endocrine or ductless glands. This means they are glands that secrete their products internally into the blood within the body, as opposed to exocrine glands that secrete to the outside via ducts, such as sweat glands. As well as glands that are exclusively endocrine in function (for example, the anterior pituitary gland) there are other organs that secrete hormones as well as performing other functions. These include the stomach, the small intestine, the skin, the liver, kidneys and the testes. All of these are made up of non-endocrine tissue with clusters of endocrine cells. The brain is an exception: it has an endocrine function but no endocrine cells.

The brain has neurosecretory neurons that function like endocrine cells. These produce neurohormones that provide an overlap or link between the nervous system and the endocrine system. It is the brain and these neuro-hormones that allow the two systems to have effects on the regulation of the other. The importance of the brain and the nervous system in the endocrine system is significant for an analysis of 'the social', as it is via the nervous system that information about the external world and other factors can influence the endocrine system. This is discussed in more detail later.

Each target cell has receptor proteins that are specific to particular hormones. Thus when a particular hormone travels by in the blood, it links up with the receptor protein in what is described as a 'lock and key' fashion. Once the hormone has been locked into the appropriate cell, it can exert its effect. Again, the constitution of the hormone affects where the receptor protein is found in the target cell: for steroid hormones, the receptors are within the cytoplasm of the cell; for polypeptides, the recep-tors are within the outer surface of the cell membrane; for thyroid hor-mones, the receptors are within the cell nucleus itself.

On arrival at the cell, the steroid hormone dissociates from its plasma carrier protein and enters the cell, attaching to the receptor protein in the cytoplasm. The combination of the hormone and the receptor protein is then 'translocated' into the nucleus of the cell. In the nucleus, this receptor protein-steroid complex is attached to an acceptor site, which 'turns on' specific genes. The genes thus activated produce nuclear RNA, which is transformed into messenger RNA (mRNA) that goes out of the nucleus into the ribosomes in the cell. In the ribosomes, the mRNA codes for new proteins to be produced. These new proteins may be enzymes that can change the metabolism of the target cell in a specific way. Thus, steroid hormones affect their target cells by stimulating genetic transcription (RNA synthesis), which then causes genetic translation (protein synthesis).

This process is slow and may take several hours. This is the major difference between the endocrine system and the nervous system (along with genes, these are the important 'messenger' systems of the body). The nervous system deals with rapid precise responses, while the endocrine system deals with activities that are slower and have long-lasting effects. The effects of the nervous system usually last for only milliseconds to seconds. The endocrine system's methods of action are slower and more complex and the effect of the action of hormones can last from minutes to days to lifetimes (in the case of growth, for example). This slowness means that the endocrine system can provide temporal control of functions – such as the menstrual cycle – that the nervous system cannot.

The endocrine system is complex. Hormones secreted by endocrine glands often have to be modified by the target cells before they can be effective. For instance, testosterone – a steroid hormone – is not effective when it leaves the gland (the testes) where it is produced. It has to be converted into more active molecules when it reaches its target cells. Target cells usually also respond to more than one type of hormone and therefore have more than one type of receptor protein. Because of this, hormones are not independent from each other but are usually affected by other hormones: either in an antagonistic fashion (where one hormone inhibits the effects of another); in a synergistic fashion (where two or more hormones work together to produce a response); or in a permissive fashion (where one hormone enhances the responsiveness of the target cell to another hormone). The sole function of some hormones is to regulate the production and secretion of other hormones. Hormones are often involved in complex interactions with each other and these interactions keep their secretion and production at required levels.

Hormones can exist in the blood for only a relatively short time, ranging from two minutes to a few hours for most hormones. Hormones are greatly diluted by the blood and must be able to exert their effect at extremely low concentrations – as low as a picogram (one millionth of a

millionth of a gram). Hormones that are not taken up and used by the
target cells are removed rapidly from the blood by the liver, deactivated
and excreted in urine. Hormones do not usually accumulate in the blood –
there are complex feedback systems that mean that when there is a certain
concentration of hormones in the blood, the endocrine gland will decrease
(or increase, as the case may be) production and secretion of that hormone.

The effects of hormones are also very concentrate-dependent. Hormones
only have their 'normal' effect when there are 'normal' (or so-called
'biological') concentrations of that hormone in the blood. If there are
pharmacological levels of hormones in the blood – due to the person taking
hormones as drugs, for example – the hormone's function may be altered.
The hormone may bind to receptor proteins of different cells and target
cells may convert the extra hormones into products with other biological
effects. Thus, for example, androgens may be turned into oestrogens under
certain circumstances of excess concentrations. Thus the administration of
large amounts of one steroid can result in the production of a significant
amount of other steroids with different effects. The responsiveness of
target cells to hormones can also be affected by the presence of other
hormones, as mentioned earlier. Sherwood writes:

> [A]lterations in the plasma concentration of a given hormone, whether caused
> by disease, administration of a hormone as a drug, or surgical removal of an
> endocrine gland, often produce widespread and unpredictable effects. Not only
> are the target tissues that are directly controlled by the hormones affected, but
> seemingly unrelated symptoms occur because of altered permissive, synergistic,
> or antagonistic effects on other hormones.
>
> *(Sherwood 1989: 643–4)*

These interactions of hormones and sensitivities to external inputs of
hormones into existing biological systems become highly pertinent in
contemporary discussions of the effects of hormones or chemicals acting
like hormones in the environment, which are discussed in Chapter 6.

The biological systems by which the amount of hormones in the blood is
regulated are most commonly negative feedback systems. Information
about the status of the hormone product is transmitted through the
blood back to the endocrine gland where it was secreted, which then
adjusts secretion accordingly. It is a negative feedback system because
the output of the system (the hormone product or effect) opposes a change
in input, i.e. when more product is made, less hormone is produced. These
systems maintain homeostasis in the body. In some cases in reproductive
endocrinology there are positive feedback systems, where the more product is made, the more hormones are produced. This leads to a building up

of product until an explosive culminating effect, such as the birth of a baby, is reached. In other cases the systems can be altered by stimuli from the external world – the neurosecretory neurons respond to stimuli received by the brain and produce an increase in hormonal secretion in the body.

It is well known that hormones do not exist at constant levels in the blood (colloquially hormones are often referred to as 'surging' or 'pumping'). Most often, hormones fluctuate in a 24 hour or circadian or diurnal cycle, in which their production oscillates over a regular one-day period. Negative feedback systems operate in conjunction with the nervous system that informs the endocrine system of changes such as light and dark. Here again the connection between the two 'messenger' systems – the nervous and the endocrine – allows fluctuation and external factors to have effects. Some rhythms of the endocrine system are longer, for example the menstrual cycle.

Central to connections between the brain and the endocrine system is the pituitary gland. This gland is situated in a cavity at the base of the brain and is connected to the hypothalamus. It is made up of two parts – the posterior and anterior pituitaries – that are functionally and anatomically distinct. In relation to sex hormones, the anterior pituitary is most important. The hypothalamus produces hormones that inhibit or increase secretion of hormones from the anterior pituitary gland. These neurohormones in turn have many influences on the secretion of hormones in other parts of the body, such as from the testes and ovaries. There are six hormones produced by the anterior pituitary which influence – are 'tropic' to – other hormones.

The pituitary gland used to be considered the 'master gland' of the body because of these six tropic hormones that are so influential in the endocrine system. However, in 1947 it was realised that these anterior pituitary hormones are in turn regulated by the neurohormones from the brain (Donovan 1988: 14–15). The search then moved backward and researchers asked what controlled the output of the neurohormones. 'Scientists now know', Sherwood writes, 'that the release of each anterior pituitary hormone is largely controlled by still other hormones produced by the hypothalamus. The secretion of these regulatory neurohormones, in turn, is controlled by a variety of neural and hormonal inputs to the hypothalamic neurosecretory cells' (Sherwood 2007: 664). Exactly what these inputs are, or how they control the secretion of the neurohormones, remains uncertain: 'Like other neurons, the neurons secreting these regulatory hormones receive abundant input of information (both neural and hormonal and both excitory and inhibitory) that they must integrate' (Sherwood 2007: 667). These neurons are connected to stress and to the emotions and 'carry information about a variety of environmental conditions' (Sherwood 2007: 668). 'The menstrual irregularities sometimes experienced by women who are emotionally upset are a common manifestation of this relationship', Sherwood (2007: 668) explains.

In this uncertain area it is possible, then, to understand how external inputs, environmental conditions, stress, emotion, the immediate metabolic state of the person and so on, might influence the production of hormones throughout the endocrine system. In general, however, physiology textbooks argue, the negative feedback systems of the endocrine system strive to maintain relatively constant rates of anterior pituitary hormone secretion. The target organ produces hormones that act in a feedback system either directly on the anterior pituitary itself, or on the hypothalamus, which then affects the pituitary. The pituitary itself, to complicate matters a little more, also seems to have a feedback system to the hypothalamus, so it can influence how much stimulating (releasing) or inhibiting neurohormone the hypothalamus produces. Other seemingly unrelated hormones can also affect the secretion of hypothalamic neurohormones. Importantly, Sherwood clearly states that it is a common phenomenon throughout the endocrine system that hormones that seem unrelated can have pronounced effects on the secretion or actions of another hormone.

So despite the tone of certainty, summary points and underlining, these physiology textbooks show that the endocrine system interacts, especially through the brain, with many other factors. Hormones are involved in fluctuating and complicated feedback systems in which each hormone has multiple and changing effects both on the metabolism of cells and thus the functions of various parts of the body and on other hormones and their functions.

The tone of certainty in textbook descriptions of the endocrine system belies the very flexibility that the system appears to have. The complex interactions of neurological and endocrine factors are important when considering how the social might enter into any activities of hormones. Spanier argues that scientific explanations of biological processes tend to understand these in isolation from the lived experience of the organism within an environment (Spanier 1995: 19–22, 98–101). This is certainly true of textbook accounts of the endocrine system. When these books move on to describe the role of hormones in the production of human bodies in development, the view that isolates biological processes from the lived experience of human beings is further undermined.

Hormones and the development of sexual differences

The foetus and the infant

Within physiological discourse there are three 'levels' of bodily difference between the sexes: genetic, gonadal and phenotypic or anatomical sex (Sherwood 1997: 705). Genetic sex is based upon a simple presence or absence of one chromosome – the Y chromosome. Gonadal sex is dependent on the existence or absence of testes and male sex hormones, and phenotypic sex is a more complicated arena. As will become clear, a key trope of scientific explanations of the role of hormones in producing sexual differences at each of these levels is that of 'absence versus presence'.

The other main trope of these discourses is the notion of development as a struggle which ends in what biologist Lewis Wolpert (1993) calls 'the triumph of the embryo'. This struggle is not one that is held to be of equal difficulty for males and females; because of the 'environment' in which embryonic and foetal development takes place (that is, within a woman's body), the struggle is said to be worse for males. For not only do males have to struggle to survive (as do females), they must struggle to resist feminisation by the mother's hormones. This notion of males struggling against the mother ties in with the absence versus presence trope in its focus on an absolute difference model of sexual difference (where each 'normal' individual is either male or female and cannot be somewhere in between). Paradoxically, this idea of male struggle also confounds the absence versus presence model, as it undoes the argument that maleness is caused only by male hormones and femaleness by the absence of these: if the male can be feminised by oestrogens, then these cannot be entirely functionless in development.

This paradox does not affect genetic sex, however. This basic level of sexual difference is seen to be a simple matter of absence or presence of the Y chromosome. Each cell in the body contains twenty-three pairs of chromosomes. During the production of sex cells, this number is halved and when fertilisation takes place the ovum and the sperm fuse and the number of chromosomes returns to forty-six, with twenty-three chromosomes coming from each parent.[3] Twenty-two of these chromosome pairs code for what are called 'general human characteristics' and other specific

---

[3] As feminist critics Spanier and Evelyn Fox Keller point out, this standard explanation ignores the fact that mothers also contribute genetic material (mitochondrial DNA) in the cytoplasm of the egg (Keller 1995: 1–42; Spanier 1995: 55–65).

traits, while the remaining pair are called the sex chromosomes. It is this pair that is either XX (female) or XY (male).

In the first four weeks of development after fertilisation, there is no evidence of this genetic difference. During the fifth week, the first sign of the reproductive organs appears – internally, the gonadal ridge is formed. This ridge grows throughout the following week and by the sixth week has 'primary sex cords' hanging from it. Externally a swelling called the genital tubercle is formed which then elongates into what is called a phallus. By the seventh week, this development of the reproductive system of the foetus is still in what is called the 'indifferent stage' because although sex organs are apparent, there is no external distinction between male and female. Up to approximately this stage, the gonads could become either male or female – being derived from the same developmental tissue, they are homologous structures.

During the seventh week gonadal specificity appears. The testes in males begin to develop under the influence of testes determining factor (TDF), which is the single gene within the Y chromosome responsible for sex determination. In females, this factor does not exist and the testes do not form. Once the testes begin to form they secrete two chemicals: testosterone and Müllerian-inhibiting factor. It is thought that a hormone secreted by the placenta causes this secretion to begin. Between days twenty-five and fifty, the embryo has two sets of ducts that could be developed into its reproductive tracts: these are the Wolffian ducts (which develop into the male reproductive system) and the Müllerian ducts (which develop into the female reproductive system). The testosterone secreted by the developing testes causes the growth of the Wolffian ducts into the male reproductive tract and begins the differentiation of the external genital swelling into the penis and scrotum. The Müllerian-inhibiting factor secreted causes the regression of the Müllerian ducts. By the beginning of the ninth week of gestation the male external genitalia are distinct and by the end of the twelfth week they are completely formed. The testes descend into the scrotal sac at the twenty-eighth week. The testosterone secretion that began at about 8 weeks reaches a peak at 12–14 weeks and then declines to very low levels by the end of twenty-one weeks. There will not be high levels of testosterone secretion again until the boy reaches puberty.

The development of a female body, as described in physiology textbooks, is based on absence or lack. As stated earlier, female genetic sex is the absence of the Y chromosome. The development of the female reproductive tract – or gonadal sex – is based on absence of the testes and the male sex hormones secreted by them. Sherwood (1989: 716) writes, 'Differentiation into a male-type reproductive system is induced by hormones secreted by the developing testes. The absence of these testicular hormones in female fetuses results in the development of a female-type reproductive system.' Neither the ovaries nor oestrogen – the most important 'female sex hormone' – are seen to be important to the development of a female reproductive tract or genitals. Female development is seen as passive: 'Note that the indifferent embryonic reproductive tissue passively develops into a female structure unless actively acted upon by masculinizing factors. In the absence of male testicular hormones, a female reproductive tract and external genitalia develop regardless of the genetic sex of the individual. Ovaries do not even need to be present for feminization of the fetal genital tissue' (Sherwood 1997: 707); 'Female sex accessory organs, therefore, develop as a result of the absence of testes rather than as a result of the presence of ovaries' (Van de Graaff and Fox 1989: 930). The explanation of this strange phenomenon concerns the mother's body, which is seen to be so high in oestrogen (secreted by her ovaries and the placenta) that if oestrogen affected foetal growth, all foetuses would become feminised.

This fear of the feminisation of the male foetus is paradoxical, as is pointed out by feminist biologist Anne Fausto-Sterling, because if female hormones play no role in foetal development why is there any fear of the feminisation of the male foetus by maternal hormones (Fausto-Sterling: 1995: 130)? In a review essay of 1985, physiologists Arthur Arnold and Marc Breedlove stated that the 'reigning dogma' was questionable, as new rodent data indicated that ovarian secretions may play some role in promoting differentiation of female neural circuits and behaviour (Arnold and Breedlove 1985: 481). '[A]t this time', they argued, 'there are sufficient data to raise important questions about the widely believed conclusion that the feminine state is merely a result of the prenatal absence of androgens or their metabolites, but these data are not completely consistent with a feminizing role for endogenous oestrogen' (Arnold and Breedlove 1985: 482).

In a more recent review published in *Behavioral and Brain Sciences*, biobehaviorists Holly Fitch and Victor Denenberg (1998) take this argument further, suggesting that ovarian oestrogens do actively produce femininity in females. In particular, Fitch and Denenberg claim that estrogens impact on the development of 'female brains' and forms of feminine behaviour in rats. Controversially, but with the support of a number of other scientists (sixteen peer commentaries are published with the article),

Fitch and Denenberg argue that the traditional emphasis on androgens in sexual differentiation and the notion of femininity as 'default' is not accurate (see also Fitch, Cowell and Denenberg 1998; Bimonte, Fitch and Denenberg 2000; Rochira *et al.* 2001). Their argument is that oestrogens' active role in producing femininity in females (the studies cited mostly concern rats, but extension to humans is also discussed), comes at a later (prenatal and postnatal) time period than exposure to androgens. Thus male foetuses can be exposed to the actions of androgens whilst females are protected from them and later, females and males can be exposed to oestrogens, with female femininity being activated and male masculinity (already activated along male pathways) not affected.[4]

Within the mainstream narrative, however, the ovaries begin to develop in the absence of male-inducing elements during the ninth week of human gestation. Without the influence of Müllerian-inhibiting factor, the Müllerian ducts develop into the uterus and the uterine tubes and the vagina and hymen form. The undifferentiated genital tubercle that in both males and females elongates and becomes the phallus, in females becomes the clitoris (in males, it becomes the penis). The labia also form and the Wolffian ducts regress without stimulation from testosterone. During this development, the female foetus also produces approximately 2 million germ cells or oocytes, a small proportion of which (approximately 400) will become ova later in her life. No new oocytes will be produced after birth. In males, in contrast, although sperm-producing cells (spermatogonia) are produced during foetal development, the production of sperm is ongoing and can continue throughout life following puberty.

These two stories describe the production of 'normal' male or female babies, but as Van de Graaff and Fox point out, 'Because an embryo has the potential to differentiate into a male or female, developmental errors can result in various degrees of intermediate sex, or hermaphroditism. A person with undifferentiated or ambiguous genitals is called a

---

[4] These arguments about the feminising role of oestrogens are linked to contemporary work on genetics. A number of the studies cited by Fitch and Denenberg (1998) investigate the activation of oestrogen receptors in various parts of the developing rodent body (see also Fitch, Cowell and Denenberg 1998; McEwan 2001). These receptors are produced by specific genes and can be studied using genetically engineered ('knock out') mice that do not have such receptors (see, for example, Hess *et al* 2001). Other researchers, for example, those at Arnold's laboratory at the University of California Los Angeles, hypothesise that genes on the sex chromosomes are expressed in brain and influence neural development directly via non-hormonal mechanisms (see www.physci.ucla.edu/physcifacultyindiv.php?FacultyKey=51. Last accessed 25 September 2006).

hermaphrodite' (Van de Graaff and Fox 1989: 950). 'Hermaphrodites' are divided into three major subgroups: the so-called true hermaphrodites who possess one testis and one ovary (i.e., one gonad of each sex); the male pseudohermaphrodites, who have testes and some aspects of the female genitalia but no ovaries; and the female pseudohermaphrodites, who have ovaries and some aspects of the male genitalia but lack testes (Fausto-Sterling 1993: 21).[5] Fausto-Sterling stresses that each of these groups is complex within itself, with individual characteristics differing widely between people so classified. The frequency of these types of hermaphroditism or intersexuality is difficult to ascertain. Fausto-Sterling quotes psychologist John Money, the most well-known specialist in this field,[6] who estimates a frequency of up to 4 per cent of births.

The causes of these various hermaphroditisms are located either at the level of genetic sex (in the case of 'true hermaphroditism'), or at the level of hormonally caused gonadal sex (for 'pseudohermaphroditism'). In the latter, the person has either the usual male XY chromosomes or the female XX chromosomes, but because of unusual hormonal levels during development of the reproductive systems, the genitals do not 'match' the chromosomes. Thus, for example, male pseudohermaphrodites, who are exposed to inadequate levels of male sex hormones, have a clitoris and vagina as well as testes and XY chromosomes. At puberty these individuals often develop breasts, but do not menstruate because they have no ovaries. Female pseudohermaphrodites have ovaries, XX chromosomes and sometimes a uterus, but also have what are called masculinised genitalia. In puberty these people can develop adult-sized penises, beards and deep voices (Fausto-Sterling 1993: 22; see also, Baker 1980).

Fausto-Sterling reports that despite the number born with these intersex characteristics, very few people in the contemporary western world are

---

[5] Bernice Hausman points out that this distinction between true and pseudohermaphrodites comes from the nineteenth-century view of hermaphrodites which held that each person had a true sex, which would be evident in the histology of the gonads. In the twentieth century, technological developments meant that the gonads of living persons could be examined and it was recognised that this notion of true gonadal sex was not sustainable. The retention of the titles 'true' and 'pseudo' hermaphrodites is a legacy of this outdated view (Hausman 1995: 77–9). The term 'intersexed' is preferred by many activists and social theorists today. I only use the term hermaphrodite in citing the textbook literature.

[6] John Money's dominance over the field of intersexed infants is very strong: 'Almost all of the published literature on intersexed infant case management has been written or cowritten by one researcher, John Money ... Even the publications that are produced independently of Money reference him and reiterate his management philosophy ... [There seems to be] a consensus that is rarely encountered in science' (Kessler 1990: 7; see also Fausto-Sterling 1995; Hausman 1995: 72–109).

left to grow to adulthood with ambiguous sexual status: 'Recent advances in physiology and surgical technology now enable physicians to catch most intersexuals at the moment of birth. Almost at once such infants are entered into a program of hormonal and surgical management so that they can slip quietly into society as "normal" heterosexual males or females' (Fausto-Sterling 1993: 22). She argues that despite the 'humanitarian' intentions, it would be better not to undertake such operations (Fausto-Sterling 1993, 2000: 45–114). In the past, Fausto-Sterling stresses, many hermaphrodites have led enjoyable lives, so there is no reason to assume that hermaphroditism is necessarily mentally unhealthy. Medical science's assumptions that there should only be two sexes and that heterosexuality is the only 'normal' sexual orientation are, she contends, what lie behind the 'humanitarian' assignment of male or female sex (Fausto-Sterling 1993, 1995, 2000).

This argument is supported by my analysis of introductory textbooks. Van de Graaff and Fox state that male pseudohermaphrodites will be sterile 'but may marry and live a normal life following hormonal therapy and plastic surgery' (Van de Graaff and Fox 1989: 950), whilst Sherwood writes, '[I]t is important to diagnose any problems in sexual differentiation in infancy. Once a sex has been assigned, it can be reinforced, if necessary, with surgical and hormonal treatment so that psychosexual development can proceed as normally as possible' (Sherwood 2007: 739). Both these quotes assume that being 'normal' is desirable, whilst the first assumes that a 'normal life' includes marriage.

Cultural theorist Bernice Hausman makes a similar argument to Fausto-Sterling, writing that surgical sex assignments are aimed more at producing heterosexual, socially unambiguous people (people who identify as either men or women) than at considering the outcomes of intervention for sexual pleasure or fertility. Hausman argues that the development of a notion of social gender as separate from biological sex has meant that surgeons feel that it is right to reconstruct bodies to fit more closely to a heterosexual two-sex model (Hausman 1995: 72–109). Important interventions have also been made in this arena by individuals diagnosed or self-identifying as intersexed. Indeed, a global network of activists now has a strong presence in the field (see, for example, Chase 1998a, 1998b, 1999; Holmes 2000).

Physiological discourses around hermaphroditism demonstrate that the role of male sex hormones in the production of sexually differentiated infant bodies is perceived as vital (see also Avila, Zoppi and McPhaul 2001). 'Normal' development of both male and female babies is understood as based on the 'correct' presence or absence of testosterone according to the chromosomal sex of the foetus. 'Abnormal' development of hermaphrodites and infants with related developmental disorders are seen to be in most cases due to unusual patterns of androgen secretion in relation to chromosomal sex. Thus, within physiological discourse, to quote pediatrician Susan Baker, there must be 'concordance' between genetic, gonadal and phenotypic sex – a concordance of presence (Y chromosome, testosterone and penis) or absence (no Y chromosome, no testosterone, and no penis) (Baker 1980: 81).

Puberty

The production of an adult body entails further complications. As Baker notes, to have true concordance as a male or female, an individual must not only have genetic, prenatal hormonal environment, gonadal and anatomical or phenotypic concordance, but also a particular postnatal hormonal environment suited to the production of their sex. 'The biological importance of this', Baker writes, 'becomes especially clear during adolescence, where elevated levels of specific female and male hormones are responsible for secondary sex characteristics. This is also the time during which the gonads assume their mature reproductive capacity' (Baker 1980: 81).

In a world that enjoys attributing sexually differentiated behaviours to the body and in particular to hormones,[7] it is perhaps surprising that between a few weeks after birth and puberty there is no difference in the blood concentrations of sex steroids (androgens and oestrogens) in boys and girls (Van de Graaff and Fox 1989: 933). During this time the two hormones produced by the anterior pituitary gland – luteinizing hormone (LH) and follicle-stimulating hormone (LSH) – are not secreted at high enough levels to stimulate any significant hormonal activity in the gonads. This 'prepubertal delay in the onset of reproductive capability', Sherwood writes, 'allows time for adequate physical and psychological maturation for the individual to handle childrearing. (This is especially important in the female, whose body must support the developing fetus.)' (Sherwood 1989: 725).[8] Such maturation also allows for ten to twelve years of cultural inscription or socialisation.

---

[7] See, for example, Steve Biddulph (1997) *Raising Boys*, discussed in detail in Chapter 3.

[8] In the 1997 and 2007 editions, Sherwood changes her mind somewhat about this, writing that this delay 'allows time for the individual to mature physically (though not necessarily psychologically) enough to handle child rearing' (Sherwood 1997: 714; 2007: 745). This change shows the importation of cultural values about mothering (specifically about psychological maturity and maternity) into this evolutionary argument.

Why, at a physiological level, puberty starts remains unknown. Some argue it is a preprogrammed event (Palmert and Boepple 2001). Others look to body weight or environmental conditions (Teilman *et al*. 2002) or examine hormonal secretions (Alonso and Rosenfield 2002). Whichever is the case, it is thought that maturational changes and decreased inhibitory mechanisms in the brain increase secretion of gonadotropin releasing hormone (GnRH) from the hypothalamus, which in turn causes increased secretion of LH and FSH from the anterior pituitary. Early in puberty GnRH is released from the brain in pulses during sleep. As puberty continues these pulses become longer until an adult pattern is established. These pulses cause increased secretion of either testosterone from the testes or oestrogen from the ovaries that causes the development of what are known as the secondary sexual characteristics.

Sherwood (1997: 702) defines the secondary sexual characteristics as 'the many external characteristics that are not directly involved in reproduction but distinguish males and females, such as body configuration and hair distribution'. 'In humans', she adds, 'the differentiating marks between males and females do serve to attract the opposite sex, but attraction is also strongly influenced by the complexities of human society and cultural behavior.' These secondary characteristics pose something of a problem for physiology and the assumptions made about the role of sexuality as species reproduction. While it is simple, within the framework of physiology textbooks, to understand the genitals, the gonads and the reproductive endocrine systems as serving the ultimate function of species survival, it is more difficult to understand bodily attributes that do not seem to contribute to this survival. For example, Van de Graaff and Fox, who define secondary sexual characteristics as 'features that are not essential for the reproductive process but that are considered to be sexual attractants', describe the problem of breasts: 'Indeed while all mammals have mammary glands and are capable of nursing, only human females have protruding breasts; the sole purpose of this characteristic, it seems, is to function as a sexual attractant' (Van de Graaff and Fox 1989: 958). It seems that it is acceptable in such textbooks to assume some sort of 'natural' or biological component to sexual attraction (and thus to reduce all sexual attraction to heterosexual attraction) for which no evidence or explanation of even possible mechanisms involved is given. The logic is this: breasts exist and are sexual attractants; therefore this must be a biological process. The social behaviours of humans becoming sexually involved with one another are thus rendered biological through their connection with parts of the body. One wonders about other secondary

sexual characteristics such as male body hair. It seems that in contemporary western culture this is not considered a sexual attractant. Must
physiology claim then that contemporary popular culture is deluded in
rejecting it as one? And further, what are we to make of the existence of
female body hair and the widespread cultural revulsion against it?

The other key event of puberty is the production of sperm and ova. The
oocytes present in the girl's body since birth begin to mature and are released
from the ovaries in a cyclical manner in ovulation. Menstruation also
begins. In boys, sperm production starts as testosterone causes the development of the seminal vesicles and the prostate gland. It is here that a
major difference between male and female hormonal physiologies is
instated: the hormonal systems established at puberty in boys involve
essentially constant testosterone secretion and continuous sperm production, while the hormonal system established in girls involves the intermit-
tent release of ova and the cyclical secretion of oestrogen.

Again, this is the pattern of 'normality'. There are individuals – those
who escaped the net of medical intervention as infants – who show unusual
or 'discordant' development at puberty. Thus, Sherwood describes how
'a masculinized genetic female with ovaries but with male-type external
genitalia may be reared as a boy until puberty, when breast enlargement
(caused by oestrogen secretion by the awakening ovaries) and lack of
beard growth (caused by lack of testosterone secretion in the absence of
testes) signal an apparent problem' (Sherwood 1997: 708). The most
famous case of this was a group of thirty-eight children from twenty-
three related families living in the Dominican Republic (Baker 1980:
89–95). At birth these children had clitoris-sized penises, incompletely
developed scrotums and sometimes external testes. They have been the
focus of much study and argument, as it has been claimed that a number of
them (nineteen, according to the famous Imperato-McGinley study cited
by Baker) were raised unambiguously as females and then became males in
puberty as their previously internal testes descended, their breasts did not
grow and their bodies generally became virilised (Baker 1980: 90). These
children have been used to argue for the importance of the biological in
development: against the view of psychologists such as John Money and
others, the 'gender identity' of these children was seen to be relatively easy
to change, once their bodies changed in puberty. That is, they quite easily
became boys. Critics of this position have argued that the children were *not*
unaffected by their unusual biologies and were in fact known by a particular name in their town, literally translated as 'penis-at-twelve' (Fausto-
Sterling 1992: 86). That these changes took place within a culture that

values men more than women may also have had something to do with the
apparent acceptability of their change to being considered male (Fausto-
Sterling 1992: 87–8).

Articulating the hormonal body

The mainstream scientific view of the role of hormones in the production
of sexually differentiated bodies is dominated by the trope of presence
versus absence. This is a dualism with a long philosophical history and
which is connected to many others such as activity/passivity and male/
female. Reliance on this dualism supports a view of sexual difference as
absolute. As was argued in Chapter 1, the science of endocrinology developed through an engagement with this model of difference. In this model,
femininity is positioned as opposite to masculinity and as therefore threatening to it. Science's understanding of the interaction between the male
foetus and the mother's hormones evidences this mode of thinking. Much
current research on the impact of environmental oestrogens on male development and sexuality also activates this model.

The active/passive distinction is also evident in endocrinology.
Maleness is seen as an active force in the story of human development –
the male foetus struggles to grow and succeeds because of his Y chromosomes and his androgen. The female foetus, on the other hand, merely
takes the default position, developing passively through lack of these
factors. As philosopher Michèle LeDoeuff writes in a discussion of contemporary psychobiology, 'From its beginnings in foetal life, "masculinity" is a thing of drama, conflict, struggle, danger, openness to influence,
relation to an Other, while "femininity" is the tranquil, immobile unfolding
of the inherent, self-closure in the same' (LeDoeuff 1989: 165).

Endocrinology's and physiology's reliance on these dualisms shows that
these sciences are not produced in cultural vacuums, but rather are implicated in and reproduce traditional notions of differences between men and
women. Paradoxically, however, their reliance on certain dichotomies
(active/passive, absence/presence) logically undercuts the ways in which
these technoscientific discourses are presumed to be structured by other
dichotomies (science/culture, objectivity/subjectivity). Endocrinology and
physiology's dependence on cultural understandings to interpret scientific
data, in other words, shows that these discourses are not 'objective' in the
sense that they are non-cultural, or designate as Haraway puts it, 'a clean
and orderly practical or epistemological space' (Haraway 1997: 68).

Further, as shown above, scientific theories about the role of the brain in the endocrine system that acknowledge and then belie the possible roles of social influences in biological processes, also undercut a simple adherence to a nature/culture, biology/social split. My aim in pointing out this complexity – in which the technoscientific discourses articulating hormonal bodies both rely on and undercut traditional dichotomies of western thought – is not to argue that these are failed or hopelessly flawed discourses. Rather, following Haraway, I am interested in thinking about how this complex set of reliance on some dichotomies and the undermining of others are part of the ways in which these particular technoscientific discourses are effective. What I want to show is that mainstream contemporary articulations of sexually differentiated hormonal bodies are constituted through a reliance on cultural understandings of sexual difference.

This mainstream scientific view of human development is open to challenge. One area in which such a challenge has been made is in the understanding of relations between the foetus and the mother. In mainstream biological descriptions, little if any attention is paid to the fact that human development is a relation between (at least) two people, that it takes place (the first few days of *in-vitro* fertilisation treatment notwithstanding) within a living woman's body. In many cases the mother of the foetus is described only as an environment, or if she is described at all it is as a potential threat, as seen above (see also Duden 1993; Hartouni 1997: 26–50). Haraway also notes this, arguing more generally that within cultural and scientific debates around foetuses, the mother 'simply disappears or re-enters the drama as an agonist' (Haraway 1992a: 312). In both legal and medical discourses, the mother-as-environment is either ignored or positioned as a possible threat to the foetus, in so far as women are seen to place their own needs above that of the foetus, for example by taking drugs during pregnancy. '[T]he woman', Haraway writes, 'is in no way a partner in an intricate and intimate dialectic of social relationality crucial to her own personhood, as well as to the possible personhood of her social – *but unlike* – internal co-actor' (Haraway 1992a: 312). Haraway argues that this understanding positions the scientist as the person who can represent the interests of the foetus, because he or she is seen as passionless and disinterested, unlike the mother. As described above, in endocrinology this understanding of the mother is also related to sex – the mother is more of a threat in hormonal terms to male than to female foetuses.

This understanding exemplifies the relation of objective scientific representation that positions nature (here, the foetus) as passive and the scientist as active. As Haraway shows, the scientist who claims to represent the foetus objectively positions it as passive in its inability to speak and thus in need of someone to represent its interests.[9] Such a positioning is dependent on the removal of the represented object from its context: 'The represented must be disengaged from surrounding and constituting discursive and non-discursive nexuses and relocated in the authorial domain of the representative' (Haraway 1992a: 312). This removal disempowers the object, renders it passive and, importantly, establishes the activity and objectivity of the scientist. '[T]he scientist is the perfect representative of nature', Haraway asserts, 'that is, of the permanently and constitutively speechless objective world. Whether he be a male or a female, his passionless distance is his greatest virtue; this discursively constituted, structurally gendered distance legitimates his professional privilege ... Nature legitimates the scientist's career' (Haraway 1992a: 312). She contrasts this relation of objective representation to one that attempts to acknowledge that activity is not limited to speech and which does not try to speak for the foetus. This alternative view acknowledges the activity of the foetus and enters into a relation of articulation with it. Such a view of scientific practice would be able to acknowledge the confounding of binary distinctions (and in fact would promote this confounding), as science would no longer be based on holding such poles apart.

A problem arises here, however, in so far as foetuses (or the body or nature) cannot represent themselves in the way of humans (that is through spoken or written language). In terms of the production of scientific knowledges, it will be humans doing the writing or speaking. The activity of the foetus or of nature, then, can only be described indirectly in discourse. The notion of articulation, however, acknowledges that scientific or other cultural discourses can never completely capture the activity of actors, whether they are human foetuses or hormones. Indeed, as Haraway argues, it is the very trickiness or 'wiliness' of actors such as hormones – their ability to escape representation's grasp – that indicates their activity. The fact that we cannot fully represent other actors does not mean that they do not exist or that they are passive. Even though we cannot represent them, she suggests:

[9] This figuration also appears in biomedical descriptions of caesarian births in which, according to Emily Martin, 'a role is constructed for the doctor to ally with the baby against the potential destruction wreaked on it by the mother's body' (Martin 1987: 64). When put next to the fact that the mother is represented as unable to do what is best for the foetus, resonances with views of anti-abortionists become alarming (Haraway 1992a: 311–12).

Perhaps we can ... 'articulate' with humans and unhumans in a social relationship, which for us is always language-mediated (among other semiotic, i.e., 'meaningful' mediations). But, for our unlike partners, well, the action is 'different,' perhaps 'negative' from our linguistic point of view, but crucial to the generativity of the collective. It is the empty space, the undecidability, the wiliness of other actors, the 'negativity,' that give me confidence in the *reality* and therefore ultimate *unrepresentability* of social nature and that make me suspect doctrines of representation and objectivity.

(Haraway 1992a: 313)

The notion of articulation, then, allows for the differences between active entities through its positing of social relationality as the central mode of relationship between the world and science. For what Haraway argues is left behind in objective representations of the world is the world itself. This is not to suggest that the world can simply be known in its activity – that we can return to the body and its 'natural' pleasures – but rather that new relations can be forged through the production of new articulations.

Feminist research about the role of the placenta provides one example of a different articulation of the relationship between mother and foetuses, one that challenges the notion of the foetus as passive. This work is discussed by biologist Hélène Rouch in an interview with philosopher Luce Irigaray. Rouch suggests that contrary to a traditional understanding of the placenta as a mechanism either of fusion (where mother and foetus become one) or of aggression (where the foetus is a parasite on the mother's body), this organ can be seen as relatively autonomous, allowing an exchange between mother and foetus that recognises the autonomy *and* interrelation of both. In relation to hormones, the placenta (which is produced by the embryo) takes over firstly from the maternal hypothalamus to control the ovaries and then from the ovaries themselves, to maintain and produce hormonal secretions needed during gestation for both the mother and the foetus. 'So what we have here', Rouch argues, 'is an organ that, although anatomically dependent upon the embryo, secretes maternal hormones that are essential during gestation when the maternal organism finds itself unable to continue its usual ovarian function owing to the state of pregnancy' (Rouch, in Irigaray 1993a: 39). Rouch uses this analysis of the placenta's role to suggest an ethical model of mother/child relations that is based neither on fusion nor violent dislocation (Irigaray 1993a: 35–44). In other words, retelling the story of the biology of the placenta allows Rouch to make an ethical, political intervention into cultural understandings of mother/foetus relations.

Messaging and articulation

Physiology textbooks attempt to describe bodily sexual differences in terms of biological processes and facts. Although they underplay or belie the role of the social in the production of sexually differentiated bodies, the writers of these books cannot provide cleanly or purely biological explanations. The social is there in theories concerning the role of the brain and in the writers' inability to produce knowledge uninfluenced by cultural understandings, despite attempts to do so. As Haraway contends, stories and facts do not maintain respectable distances in technoscience: the writers of physiological textbooks cannot keep stories of sexual difference, of sexual antagonism, or evolutionary heterosexual attraction, out of their epistemological space.

The mainstream view of science as objectively representing nature – of separating facts and stories – is dependent on the maintenance of binary oppositions and relies especially on positioning nature as passive and the scientist as active. Haraway's notion of articulation is an important alternative to this understanding. In its figuration of technoscience as interaction between human and non-human actors, articulation forms a connection with this book's theme of messaging. Both notions invoke communication between the social and biological; specifically, they configure two- (or more-) way communications that constitute both biological and social actors as active and that are thus disruptive of modern technoscientific configurations of activity and passivity. These forms of communication involve the 'promiscuous cohabit[ing]' by stories and facts of the material and epistemological spaces constituting scientific knowledges and practices. As in the example of foetal masculinisation and the potential for the mother's hormones to 'swamp' the male foetus, stories and facts intermingle quite inextricably in discourses of endocrinology.

Although in modern understandings of technoscience this intermingling would be seen as a deficiency or problem (a failure to adhere correctly to the scientific method), the aim of describing technoscience as articulation, or figuring the actions of hormones in the production of sexually differentiated bodies as messaging, is not to provide a negative critique but rather to elaborate a convincing analysis of how scientists engage with nature or the world. Haraway's notion of articulation figures the actions of scientists as an interaction with non-human actors or as a 'social relationship' (Haraway 1992a: 313). My notion of messaging focuses on the actions of specific non-human actors (sex hormones) and likewise figures these as partaking in social relationships with other actors, both human and non-human. The nature of this social relationship is highly complex and takes place in particular material-semiotic spaces and at specific times. As this chapter has demonstrated, in contemporary physiology and endocrinology texts, hormones message sexual difference both materially (in their actions in cells) and discursively. As in the case of male body hair (which is supposed to be a sexual attractant), hormones' material actions in cells are described as producing inevitable social meanings. Hormones thus convey the freight of cultural understandings of sexual difference and its supposedly 'natural' connection to heterosexuality and reproduction in technoscientific explanations of specific bodily differences. In my (reconfigured) understanding of hormonal actions as messaging, hormones are not carriers of already-established or 'natural' differences, but rather are engaged in social and therefore political articulations or interactions with humans that in specific times and places produce particular versions of sexual difference. This version of hormones as messengers of sex means, then, that these actions can be changed, revised, understood differently, and I have given some examples of how this might be achieved in this chapter. Chapter 3, which moves into the psychological sciences and investigates the ways in which hormones message there, provides further elaboration of this argument through new examples.

3

Activating sexed behaviours

> As we have long suspected, the minds of men and women are very
> different – and here at last is the proof.
>
> (*Daily Mail*, back-cover blurb on Baron-Cohen 2004)

Since their 'discovery' in the early twentieth century, sex hormones have
played a strong role in the explanation of sex differences in human and
other animal behaviours. Within the contemporary sciences of biological
psychology and behavioural endocrinology, they are attributed powers to
produce sex differences in behaviours such as children's play and adult
sexuality. In popular scientific literature, hormonal differences are also
thought to demonstrate that women are better suited than men to childrearing, and to underlie the sexes' different capacities for other types of
work. British psychiatrist Simon Baron-Cohen, author of *The Essential
Difference* (2004), for example, describes the ways in which prenatal hormonal environments create what he calls male or female brains.[1] The male
brain, created by *in-utero* exposure to testosterone, has skills in system-
atising, which is 'the drive to analyse, explore and construct a system'
(Baron-Cohen 2004: 3). Female brains, on the other hand, excel at empathi-
sing, which refers to 'the drive to identify another person's emotions and
thoughts and to respond to them with an appropriate emotion' (Baron-
Cohen 2004: 2). These hormonally based drives lead 'naturally' to particular jobs:

> People with the female brain, make the most wonderful counsellors, primary-
> school teachers, nurses, carers, therapists, social workers, mediators, group
> facilitators or personnel staff. Each of these professions requires excellent

---

[1] Somewhat unconvincingly, Baron-Cohen (2004: 8–9) insists that these brain types do not
necessarily map onto biological sex.

empathizing skills. People with the male brain make the most wonderful scientists, engineers, mechanics, technicians, musicians, architects, electricians, plumbers, taxonomists, catalogists, bankers, toolmakers, programmers or even lawyers. Each of these professions requires excellent systematizing skills.

(Baron-Cohen 2004: 185)

Needless to say, Baron-Cohen does not comment on the differential pay rates or prestige of these professions, nor give any historical account of their development. His argument is entirely biological: these differences are linked to exposure to sex hormones *in utero*. In a publication providing more technical information on the studies of hormones in amniotic fluid on which much of the argument of *The Essential Difference* is based, Baron-Cohen and colleagues (2004) discuss a finding that parents speak more often to girl babies than to boy babies, and that girls engage in more eye contact:

One possibility is that the propensity of girls to engage in this dyadic interaction has its foundations in prenatal biology, and that, if parents are talking to girls more, it is because girls elicit this by their relative precocity of social-communicative development. This idea is supported by the biological findings of our experiment.

(Baron-Cohen et al. 2004: 89)

Social differences in parenting behaviour, in this view, are elicited by babies' biology, rather than being culturally inflected. It is these differences that, according to Baron-Cohen, ultimately determine the sexual division of labour in contemporary societies.

This kind of scientific work is popular and is frequently reported in the international press. Given this, it is important that feminist responses to it are substantial. Whilst critiques of biological reductionism in the explanation of sex differences in human and other animal behaviour are well established within feminist thought,[2] there are two central reasons that more specific attention needs to be paid to the positive theorisation of the role of biology in the production of sexed behaviours. Firstly, on many occasions, scientists *do* attempt to account for the social in their work (that is, they do not provide accounts that are entirely reductionist in a biological sense); this work also needs feminist examination. Secondly, theoretical discussions within feminism (such as those described in the Introduction) demonstrate that it is difficult, if not impossible, to entirely dismiss the role of the biological in the production of sex differences. It remains inadequate – theoretically and politically – for feminism simply to reject the biological (for similar arguments see Wilson 1998, 2004; Hird

---

[2] See, for example, Bleier 1984; Fausto-Sterling 1992; Spanier 1995; Birke 1999.

2004). Instead, this chapter attempts to theorise the biological in its powerful and historically specific hormonal instantiations without being reductionist. To do this, it works with critical technoscientific research into animal behaviour and with contemporary feminist theories of biology and sex, as well as providing critical readings of historical and current technoscientific theorising.

Hormones and 'the organ of behaviour'

How do the technoscientific disciplines of behavioural endocrinology and biological psychology explain the connections between the brain, the biological body and human behaviour? What is the role of hormones in this understanding, insofar as it relates to sex differences?

The most simple view – what biologist David Crews calls the classical view – is biologistic. It argues that 'all somatic sexual dimorphisms, including brain, and hence behaviour, result from gonadal hormone production that begins after morphological differentiation of the gonad' (Crews 1988: 332). In this view, brain and behavioural factors derive directly from sexed bodily differences. Thus, for example, studies are made of the sexuality of rats, whereby early androgen levels are manipulated and later changed patterns of sexual behaviour noted. The theory is that androgen causes masculine behaviour and its absence causes feminine behaviour. As physiologist Bernard Donovan states, 'This idea can be traced back to classical studies [in 1959] of the hormonal control of the differentiation of the genital tract, for when pregnant guinea-pigs were injected with androgen the genitalia of the female offspring were masculinized and they showed an increase in male-type mounting behaviour and aggressiveness' (Donovan 1988: 236). In later research, male rats were deprived of androgens by castration or by treatment with anti-androgenic drugs, which was seen to result in the 'later manifestation of the female pattern of lordosis [the female position adopted during mating, which is used as the yardstick of feminine sexual behaviour in rats] after priming with oestrogen and progesterone' (Donovan 1988: 236). Thus a simple causal chain was established between the sexual behaviour of animals such as guinea pigs and rats and their hormonally sexually differentiated bodies.

This research created leads into more compelling questions of human sexuality. In 1988, feminist theorists of science Ruth Doell and Helen Longino described the increasing attempts, since the early 1970s, to develop theories of human behaviour based on extrapolation from these animal studies. Using the linear model applied in animal studies (the one-way causal model where chromosomes cause gonads, which cause hormones, which cause behaviours), human behaviour is studied as an effect of prenatal hormonal input: 'The human brain is treated largely as a black box with prenatal hormonal input and later behavioural output. The implication is that the effect of prenatal hormone exposure can be either quantitatively assessed as contributing a specific amount to the end result, or that it is, by itself, determinative of that result' (Doell and Longino 1988: 59). In this simplistic model, differences between humans and non-human animals are largely erased and the influence of the social on behaviour is reduced to little or nothing. Often-cited producers of this type of work include psychologists John Money, Anke Ehrhardt and Heino Meyer-Bahlburg, all of whom have studied the behavioural patterns of 'special' human populations exposed to unusual levels of hormones *in utero*.

'Normal' human populations are also studied in this way. As it is not possible in these populations to know the levels of hormones to which infants were exposed *in utero*, measurements of current levels of hormones are taken. This is followed by measurement of whatever behaviour is being observed and the proposition of a causal link. Such a proposition extrapolates correlations to causes. Marianne Hassler, for example, studies the 'effect' of testosterone (T) on musical ability, finding 'that an optimal T level may exist for the expression of creative musical behaviour' (Hassler 1992: 55). Many assumptions underlie this work: Hassler admits to assuming that 'current T levels can be looked at as a component of a relatively enduring biochemical system which has been organized during prenatal and/or perinatal brain development under the influence of androgens and/or oestrogens' (Hassler 1992: 66). She assumes, in other words, that the brain is set up during the prenatal and/or perinatal period in a male or female way, and levels of adult hormone can be used as an indicator of this set-up. She rejects suggestions that the musical ability she finds may have more to do with environmental influences than T levels by citing examples of children from musical families where one child became a musician and others did not (for example, Mendelssohn) (Hassler 1992: 67). Hassler considers this sufficient argument to establish the causal importance of T levels and 'male-type' or 'female-type' brains and endocrine systems. This view of what is non-biological – the idea everyone in one family has the same experience of 'the social' – is absurdly limited.

As Doell and Longino note, the linear model problematically figures the brain as a passive biological entity. In much literature on human and other animal behaviour, however, *some* attention is given to the complexities of the brain and its relation to hormones and to the social.[3] Despite this, Doell and Longino argue that this does not mean the abandonment of the linear model of causation for many scientists (Doell and Longino 1988: 60). References to the importance of the social are often made and then forgotten. In cases where closer attention is paid, scientists acknowledge the brain as a meeting point between the endocrine system and 'input' from the external world. Throughout this literature there are many different frameworks of understanding this relation between the body, brain and the world, most of which involve a division of processes or functions into those that are more biological (more directly caused by hormones) and those that are more social. This process of division shows that these theories maintain a reliance on the social/biological distinction.

The work of medical psychologists John Money and Anke Ehrhardt are good examples of this. In 1955 Money suggested that there is a fundamental difference between gender identity or role (sense of self as male or female) and sex dimorphic behaviours. Gender identity, he found, was not dependent on gonadal sex, but rather was determined by rearing. Thus a child born with complete androgen insensitivity who was genetically male but raised as a girl had a female gender identity that was stable and difficult to change, even when bodily changes in puberty made her body seem male (Ehrhardt 1984: 42–4). Ehrhardt, a colleague of Money's, follows this view in her work on sexed behaviours. She agrees that gender identity may be socially caused, but argues on the other hand that sexed behaviours such as playing with dolls and rough-and-tumble play have a biological (prenatal hormonal) basis (Ehrhardt and Meyer-Bahlburg 1981; Ehrhardt 1984). Sexual orientation is further split off, as is cognitive behaviour such as performance on cognitive tests. These latter two are not seen by Ehrhardt to be hormonally caused, although she suggests that future evidence may prove that they are (Ehrhardt and Meyer-Bahlburg 1981; Ehrhardt 1984).[4]

Other scientists give more prominence to the role of the brain, conceptualising behaviour as a result of a complex brain/body interaction. June Machover Reinisch, Mary Ziemba-Davis and Stephanie A. Sanders, for

[3] Whilst the articles discussed here represent important strands of research into sex hormones and brain development, this chapter does not attempt a comprehensive appraisal of the field of neuropsychology. Rather, the research is used as evidence of particular modes of understanding the social/biological distinction prominent within behavioural endocrinology and biological psychology. For a more comprehensive feminist analysis of neuropsychology, see Wilson 1998.

[4] Ehrhardt's work since the mid-1980s has focused on issues relating to HIV/AIDS and sexuality, rather than sex differences.

example, acknowledge that much research has demonstrated the importance of the social in the production of human behaviour. Thus they make a claim for 'biological potentiality' rather than biological determinism. Reinisch and colleagues 'have conceptualized the complex interaction between organismic and environmental factors in the development of sex differences in human behaviour as the "multiplier effect"' where from birth to adulthood (prenatally) hormonally caused differences in the brain affect the sensations and perceptions received by the brain and the cognitions produced, and establish 'behavioural predispositions' that cause 'slightly different' male or female behaviours (Reinisch *et al.* 1991: 214). These 'slightly different' behaviours, they argue, are then encouraged or discouraged by caretakers and others. This encouragement increases the influence of the social on behaviour. As puberty is reached, differences are further 'augmented' and during adult reproductive years the differences between men and women are at a maximum. 'As humans age', they go on to claim, 'perhaps because role expectations become less divergent, there appears to be a tendency for both sexes to become more androgynous and therefore more similar, resulting in the relative reduction of sex differences among older adults' (Reinisch *et al.* 1991: 214).

Despite their adherence to this 'multiplier effect' model, which takes into account the social via the insistence on brain differences between the sexes and the reinforcement of these through 'social roles', Reinisch and colleagues, in reviewing nineteen studies of the behavioural patterns of children and adults exposed to 'prenatal hormone environments that were atypical for their sex', end up ignoring the effects of the social on human behaviour (Reinisch *et al.* 1991: 215). They position the role of the social as a possible confounding factor that can be separated surprisingly easily from a study of the role of biology (hormones):

> By studying the effects of prenatal exposure to these exogenous hormones, insight may be gained into the role of prenatal endogenous hormones in the development of behavioural differences both within and between the sexes. However, because the role of prenatal hormonal exposure in the development of human behavioural sex differences is potentially confounded by society's differential treatment of male and female individuals, this review focuses on making comparisons within a given sex. The demonstration of within-sex behavioural differences attenuates the confound between prenatal hormonal contributions and environmental influences on the development of sexually dimorphic behaviour.
>
> *(Reinisch et al. 1991: 215)*

So by separating the sexes, everything becomes strangely simple. Reinisch and colleagues erase the effect of culture through their acknowledgement of the differential treatment of boys and girls: yes, culture exists, they say, but it is relevant only insofar as it affects the sexes differentially. Thus, if we only compare males with males and females with females, the 'confound' inflicted by the social will be 'obviated' (Reinisch *et al.* 1991: 271). This assumption that the social treatment of all the members of one sex is identical is insupportable.

In their review, Reinisch and colleagues examine studies of the behaviour of adults or children who have been exposed *in utero* to atypical patterns of hormones. These people's behaviours are compared to those of others who were not exposed to such 'environments'. Comparisons are made according to a scale of masculinity and femininity: with the help of the articles reviewed and with four psychologists, Reinisch and colleagues classify the sets of behaviours studied into masculine or feminine behaviours. They then indicate if the people exposed to atypical hormone levels are masculinised, defeminised, feminised, or demasculinised, according to whether or not they exhibit behaviours nominated as either masculine or feminine. Masculinisation and feminisation are said to occur when the subject shows more of a clearly masculine or feminine behaviour. Demasculinisation or defeminisation is said to occur when there is a decrease in a masculine or feminine behaviour, but which is not necessarily seen to be a swing to its 'opposite'. Unsurprisingly, behaviours seen to be feminine include 'interest in playing with dolls', 'interest in appearance and hairstyles' and 'interest in marriage and maternalism', while masculine behaviours included 'rough-and-tumble play', 'aggression', 'interest in watching sports on TV' and 'participation in sports'. Homo- and heterosexuality are also figured here: for young male subjects, preferring to play with boys is rated as masculine, whereas playing with girls is rated as feminine. In late adolescence and adulthood, however, 'this assumption was not made' (Reinisch *et al.* 1991: 226). That these very categories reflect the social in historically specific ways is not of interest to Reinisch and colleagues. They simply note the hormonal influences on the infant, observe its later behaviour, noting whether there has been a masculinisation or feminisation, and then nominate this change as biological.

Logically, this process means that Reinisch and colleagues must ultimately claim either that there is some sort of biological force that produces 'playing with dolls' and 'interest in watching sports on TV' (which is nonsensical), or that there is some (biological?) intermediary between the body/brain and these culturally influenced behaviours. This intermediary is presumably what they call 'behavioural predispositions' (Reinisch *et al.* 1991: 271), but we are given no information as to what these actually are.

We know there are hormones and there are social behaviours that can be socially rated as masculine or feminine, but there is still no explained connection between the two. In quoting Stephen Gould – 'Humans are animals, and everything we do is constrained, in some sense, by our biology' (quoted in Reinisch *et al.* 1991: 213–14) – Reinisch and colleagues reveal their assumed position. They prove nothing and yet claim to have demonstrated an important role for prenatal hormones in child and adult behaviour. All they have shown is that people who were exposed to various hormones during foetal development occasionally show different scores on tests of stereotypical social behaviours. Nothing is demonstrated (but much is assumed) about the role of biology in the lives of their human subjects.[5]

When technoscience looks at the role of hormones in the establishment of sexually differentiated behaviours, questions of homo- and heterosexuality are never far behind. Cheryl McCormick, Sandra Witelson and Edward Kingstone, for example, situate their study of the biological factors in the aetiology of homosexuality within a growing search for such factors, which they claim is 'partly due to results of experimental work of the last few decades which show that much of the sexual behaviour of non-human animals is driven by sex hormones' (McCormick *et al.* 1990: 69). McCormick and colleagues argue that adult hormone levels will be unlikely to provide an explanation for sexual orientation and so it would be more profitable to look to the brain, which they call 'the organ of behaviour' (McCormick *et al.* 1990: 69). They state that 'to a certain extent, sexual differentiation of the brain is independent of the sexual differentiation of other parts of the body ... Thus, one may predict neural differences between homosexuals and heterosexuals without expecting other biological differences' (McCormick *et al.* 1990: 70). Their findings (which focus on the incidence of left-handedness in homo- and heterosexual men and women in order to indicate levels of brain hemispheric lateralisation),[6] they argue, support the notion that prenatal neuroendocrine events

---

[5] This approach to studying the behaviour of children has been taken up in more recent years by scientists interested in discerning the effects of endocrine disrupting chemicals on humans (see, for example, Ferguson 2002; Vreughenhil *et al.* 2002). This work is discussed in Chapter 6.

[6] A self-report 12-item questionnaire was used to ascertain the hand preference of 32 homosexual women and 38 homosexual men and the levels of left-hand preference were compared to previously measured levels of handedness in a general population sample (N = 2322). The homosexual women were found to have higher prevalence of left-hand preference, a result that is used to argue for 'atypical pattern of hemispheric lateralization in this group' (McCormick *et al.* 1990: 2). Homosexual men did not differ from the general population

are 'a factor' in the development of human sexual orientation and that the mechanisms associated with sexual orientation differ between the sexes (McCormick *et al.* 1990: 69). In this work the brain is not figured as a 'black box' but more as a neuroendocrine controller. Prenatal hormones are seen to affect the brain and thus behaviour, in a way that is separate from their effect on the body via gonads (measured in hormone levels in the blood).

This more complicated idea – that the brain itself is sexually differentiated by hormones in a separate process to the sexual differentiation of the gonads and thus the body in general – is taken up by many scientists. One year after this research on homosexuality, Witelson (1991) published a review of studies of sex differences in human brain organisation and behaviour. In this review she works through research concerning different neurological areas and finds evidence of sex differences in each. These differences she attributes to prenatal and perinatal hormonal action. 'Research has demonstrated', she asserts,

> that the brain is a sexually differentiated organ, that is, that fetal and perinatal sex hormones have organizational effects on brain structure and also have subsequent activational effects on the brain ... Such results have led to hypotheses of the role of sex-related biological factors leading to the variation in human brain function and behaviour, but the specific relationships and mechanisms remain to be delineated.
>
> *(Witelson 1991: 132)*

In other words, she reports correlations between certain brain differences and types of behaviours, but can only assume causal relationships. Throughout the article Witelson states that sex differences in various parts of the brain could affect particular behaviours and so ends up concluding that there is a biological basis of behavioural and cognitive differences between the sexes and between homosexuals and heterosexuals (Witelson 1991: 148). The implications of this finding do not disturb her, as she hands over responsibility to others: 'The challenge *to society*', she

---

sample. Problems with this study include low subject numbers and the fact that homosexual subjects were recruited from 'a local homophile organization' and therefore may have had many social factors in common. The logic of the discussion is also odd: McCormick and colleagues argue that from their results 'one would expect' that 4 per cent of left-hand-preferring women would be homosexual and 1 per cent of right-hand-preferring women to be homosexual. Ninety-six per cent of left-handed-preferring women, in other words, would not be homosexual. As a causal explanation for female homosexuality then, brain hemispheric lateralisation (as demonstrated by hand preferences) seems very weak indeed. For further critical evaluation of studies regarding hand preference and brain lateralisation, see Rogers 1999: 103–18.

asserts, 'is to accept, respect, and effectively use the neural diversity among human beings' (Witelson 1991: 148, emphasis added).

This notion of the brain as neuroendocrine controller in both gender and sexual orientation retains currency in more recent scientific research.[7] In a review published in *Gynaecological Endocrinology*, for example, D. F. Swaab (2004: 301) enthusiastically affirms this model, writing that 'male sexual differentiation of the human brain is thought to be determined in the two first periods during which sexually dimorphic peaks in gonadal hormone levels are found – during gestation and the perinatal period, while from puberty onwards, sex hormones alter the previously organized neuronal systems ("activating effects")'. 'It is', he adds, 'the prenatal testosterone surge that is most important for the development of gender identity' (Swaab 2004: 301). Affirmative of this neurological model, Swaab's work is explicitly pitted against the suggestion that there might be social explanations for gender identity, sexual orientation or even transsexualism: 'Solid evidence for the importance of postnatal social factors is lacking', he asserts (Swaab 2004: 301).

In all of these theories, the claim to account for the role of the social in the production of sexually differentiated behaviours is false. In each, the social is reduced to simplistic ideas of what happens in families (that everyone in the same family is treated equally) or in society (that all members of the same sex are treated equally). Notions of racial, class or cultural differences are ignored, as is the wealth of feminist and other work on the complexity of the social and its effects on human embodiment. This simplistic understanding of the social allows these writers to strengthen their claims about the role of biology (hormones) in the production of behaviours. They claim to have controlled for, or to have examined the social and then to have found that the biological is more important.

Scientific challenges to the biological/social distinction: animal studies

In the view of these scientists, biology can be separated from the social. The biological body is understood as established during development and is thought to remain quite stable throughout a life. The brain in particular is conceptualised as a relatively static entity. In contrast to this mainstream

---

[7] See, for example, Hines 1998; Neave and Menaged 1999; Wilson 1999; Slabbekoorn *et al.* 2000; Swaab 2004.

idea, other scientists stress the flexibility and responsiveness of the brain to the external world, arguing that the human brain is affected and changed by the external world, not just by prenatal endocrine events. Physiologist Lesley Rogers, for example, writes:

> The brain is able to learn and in so doing its biochemistry and cellular structure are changed. Thus environmental influences alter its storage and capacity to process information, and thus can affect the course of brain development ...
> This is often forgotten in discussions of brain structure and function. The brain is seen as a controller determining behaviour, and often insufficient attention is paid to feedback of behaviour and other environmental influences on brain development and function. Although it is possible that sex hormones can influence brain development, it is equally possible that environmental factors can do the same.
>
> *(Rogers 1988: 49)*

This means that there can be another interpretation of the correlations found between types of brains and certain behaviours discussed above: behaving in certain ways can change the brain. As Rogers argues, 'the effect of testosterone on the brain does not occur in the absence of environmental influences and it cannot be considered in separation from these' (Rogers 1988: 51). According to Rogers, the human brain remains plastic throughout life, thus no correlation can be assumed to be caused by hormones or genes (Rogers 1999: 111). The challenge to scientists, she states, is to design research that can investigate the simultaneous and perhaps inseparable effects of hormones and the environment on the development of brain and behaviour.

There are many studies of non-human animals that show that brain development and production of sexed behaviours is dependent on social environment. Rogers' work describes the role of light on the outside of the egg for the development of chicks' brains. Her studies demonstrate that, rather than being genetically or hormonally determined, lateralised brain development and subsequent sex differences in chicks' food-seeking behaviours are also influenced by this light (Bradshaw and Rogers 1993: 54–9; Rogers 1998; Rogers 1999: 111–15). Sex hormones interact with light stimulation to produce sex differences.

Psychologist Celia Moore comes to a similar conclusion in her extensive work with rats. In contrast to the classical studies discussed above, Moore demonstrates that hormonal development and adult sexual behaviour in rats is partially dependent on maternal behaviour when they were pups. In a series of studies, Moore and colleagues have shown that because of a scent they excrete male pups receive more anogenital licking from their mothers than do female pups.[8] When they do not receive this licking (for instance when dams are prevented from smelling the pups or when they are stressed during pregnancy), rats do not display typical sexual behaviour in adulthood (Moore 1984; Moore and Power 1986; 1992). Female rats treated with male hormones and receiving more licking than others display atypical sexual behaviour as adults. As Moore states, these pieces of evidence show that maternal behaviour mediates the actions of sex hormones. Her studies 'fail ... to support generally accepted views that early hormones affect behaviour through direct effects on brain differentiation ... Hormones coact and interact with other factors throughout development ... Hormone-based sources of sex differences may be located throughout the body and in the social surround' (Moore quoted in Rogers 1988: 46).[9]

Other animal studies also show the essential role of the environment in producing so-called hormonally caused behaviour: male cichlid fish have to have physical contact with other males in order to be hormonally able to reproduce (Francis *et al.* 1993; Fox *et al.* 1997); in some birds sight of the male bird or hearing his song causes the female bird's ovaries to secrete hormones and accelerate egg growth (West, White and King 2003: 51–89); and female rhesus monkeys are unable to have sex or to care for their young if they are raised in isolation from other monkeys (Haraway 1989: 231–43). In humans, testosterone secretion in men can be suppressed under extreme stress and elevated through sport and sexual fantasy (Rogers 1999: 75–6).

Other research shows that the social and physical environment of certain animals can cause a complete change in sex and thus in sexed behaviour. David Crews' work on reptiles, for example, demonstrates that in some species, gonadal differentiation is determined during embryogenesis as a consequence of environment (external temperature), rather than as a result of chromosomes (Crews 1988: 328–9). Other animals, including some types of fish, are hermaphroditic and change sex according to their social environment (for example, the disappearance of a dominant male or female) either only once or repeatedly (Crews 1994: 100–1). Still other animal species are not sexually differentiated at all (they are all females), but reproduce asexually in parthenogenesis (self-cloning). This does not mean that these animals (for example, species of whiptail lizards)

---

[8] See Moore 1984; Moore and Power 1992; Moore and Dou 1996; Moore *et al.* 1997.
[9] Rogers (1999: 109–11) also reports studies showing that handling of rat pups by humans after birth influences brain development when testosterone is also present (i.e., in males or if females are injected with testosterone). These results also support the contention that hormonal effects are entwined with social interactions in the production of sex differences.

do not engage in sexual behaviour. They engage in behaviour that is identical to the mating behaviour of sexually differentiated species, but in which the females take turns to act male or female parts. This sexual interaction is believed to cause the females to lay more eggs than they would if they were alone (Crews 1994: 101).[10]

Crews uses this research to argue against the simplistic theory that chromosomes cause gonadal sex, which via hormones causes masculine or feminine characteristics and sexual behaviours. In particular, he argues against the concomitant notion (discussed in Chapter 2) that males are the 'organised' or differentiated sex and females the 'default' sex (that is, that the action of androgens causes males to develop, while females are produced in the absence of androgens). Key to his argument is evidence that both of the so-called female hormones – oestrogen and progesterone – may play an active role in male sexuality. In some species, including humans and rats, testosterone is converted to oestrogen in the brain and activates both male and female copulatory behaviours (Crews 1994: 103; see also Fitch and Denenberg 2000; Alonso and Rosenfield 2002). As Rogers states:

> Males secrete the so-called 'female' sex hormone, oestrogen, and females secrete the 'male' sex hormone, testosterone. Indeed, some females have higher plasma levels of testosterone than do some males. In the brain, where sex hormones are meant to cause sex differences in behaviour, the distinction between the sexes becomes even less distinct. There are no known sex differences in the binding of oestrogen in the hypothalamic area of the brain, let alone binding at higher levels of brain organisation; and testosterone must be converted to oestrogen intracellularly before it can act on neurones.
>
> *(Rogers 1988: 44)*

As both Rogers and Crews point out, then, animals do not form entirely male or female brains and, in animals such as rats, female nerve circuits are not lost in males but can be activated by hormone administration (Rogers 1988: 45; Crews 1994). It is the interacting roles of the social, environmental and hormonal, they argue, that cause any particular male or female behaviour in animals.

These examples of the interaction of the social and the biological in non-human animals are useful challenges to the biological psychological theories outlined earlier, because they demonstrate that even in supposedly

---

[10] Crews' interpretation of these behaviours has been the subject of controversy within major scientific journals. For a discussion of this controversy and an analysis of Crews' diverse writing practices, see Myers 1990.

'simple' animals such as rats and chicks (animals that are used as models in these sciences to argue for biological causality of behaviours) and lizards, birds and fish, sexually differentiated behaviours are not directly caused by biology. Even though hormones are understood to play an important role in the production of these behaviours, this role cannot be theorised in isolation from the animal's physical environment and its interactions with other animals. If the behaviour of 'simple' animals is not caused biologically, then how can a legitimate claim be made in relation to humans, who are perceived within these sciences as more complicated and complex than other animals?

Feminist challenges to the biological/social distinction: the lived body

Alterity is the very possibility and process of embodiment: it conditions but is also a product of the pliability or plasticity of bodies which makes them other than themselves, other than their 'nature', their functions and identities.
(Grosz 1994: 209)

Contemporary feminist theories of the body provide tools for a critique and rethinking of the biological/social distinction evident in biological psychology and behavioural neuroendocrinology. This section outlines this work, with a particular focus on that of philosopher Elizabeth Grosz, in order to develop a more complex notion of the interrelation of the social and biological.

Grosz's book *Volatile Bodies* (1994) forms part of an important body of feminist theory stemming from the 1980s in the wake of poststructuralist analyses of psychoanalysis. As discussed in the Introduction, this body of work – which also includes Judith Butler's *Gender Trouble* (1990), *Bodies That Matter* (1993) and *Undoing Gender* (2004), Moira Gatens' *Imaginary Bodies* (1996) and Rosi Braidotti's *Metamorphoses* (2002) and *Transpositions* (2006) – problematises the distinction made in earlier feminist thinking between sex and gender, in which sex was a biological substrate and gender an externally produced social interpretation. Each of these writers theorises the body as an entity that disrupts the social/biological distinction and is active in the production of gender and sexual differences.

In opposition to the idea that the biological body exists independently of representations of it (which can be objectively made by technoscience), these theorists argue that representations and understandings of the body

participate in the very constitution of bodies. Grosz, for example, writes in
the introduction to *Volatile Bodies*:

> I will deny that there is the 'real', material body on one hand and its various
> cultural and historical representations and cultural inscriptions on the other.
> It is my claim ... that these representations and cultural inscriptions quite
> literally constitute bodies and help produce them as such.
>
> *(Grosz 1994: x)*

As outlined in the Introduction, Butler makes a similar claim about sexed
bodies, arguing that these are materialised through the repeated performative social practices that constitute gender.

Importantly, neither Grosz nor Butler suggest that bodies are utterly
constituted by language or have no biological content. Butler clearly states
that there are 'undeniable materialities' (including 'hormonal and chemical composition') pertaining to the body, but suggests that there are no
clear boundaries that divide these materialities from cultural interpretations of them (Butler 1993: 66–7). This notion of the inseparability of the
biological and social in the production of sexed bodies is also espoused by
Grosz: '[T]he interimplication of the natural and the social or cultural
needs further investigation', she writes, 'the hole in nature that allows
cultural seepage or production must provide something like a natural
condition for cultural production; but in turn the cultural too must be
seen in its limitations, as a kind of insufficiency that requires natural
supplementation' (Grosz 1994: 21). Grosz's suggestion here is to problem-
atise the strict division between nature and culture or biology and society
and to think of these terms instead as somehow mutually dependent, with
each requiring the other for its existence. Biology is seen to be endlessly
open to cultural intervention, but nevertheless to retain some existence: it
is the body which then becomes 'the threshold or borderline concept that
hovers perilously and undecidably at the pivotal point of the binary pairs'
(Grosz 1994: 23).

This notion of the body as a threshold is further explicated in Grosz's
understanding of sexual difference. Rejecting a social-constructivist view
of the body as a passive and neutral recipient of social inscription, and yet
also refusing any simple biologistic view of 'obvious' sexual differences,
means that sexual difference must be rethought along the same lines as the
body itself. Grosz writes:

> I am reluctant to claim that sexual difference is purely a matter of the inscription
> and codification of somehow uncoded, absolutely raw material, as if these
> materials exert no resistance or recalcitrance to the processes of cultural

inscription. This is to deny a materiality or a material specificity and determinateness to bodies. It is to deny the postulate of a pure, that is, material difference. It is to make them infinitely pliable, malleable. On the other hand, the opposite extreme also seems untenable. Bodies are not fixed, inert, purely genetically or biologically programmed entities that function in their particular ways and in their determinate forms independent of their cultural milieu and value.

(Grosz 1994: 190)

Again Grosz argues that the problem here is the attempt to separate the biological and the social into two distinct categories. Instead she suggests that each side is necessary and limits the other in ways that can never be set in advance, but that nonetheless have significant effects. From this point of view, sexual difference, although always overwritten with cultural values, must contain some sort of biological dimension, a dimension that can be seen as a materiality that makes developments possible. Sexual difference is not a matter of preexisting categories with set contents, but is an interval or gap – a radical difference – between the sexes' experiences and knowledges. It does not fit clearly into the dualism of nature and culture (Grosz 1994: 208–9; see also Grosz 2005: 171–83).

In these theorists' view of the nature/culture distinction, one side of the dualism always operates as a limit for the other side. Although it is argued that such limits are never knowable in advance, there is a tendency to emphasise the flexibility of the social in contrast to the fixity of the biological. Butler, for example, tends to place stronger emphasis on the flexibility of gender than the materialities of sex in her readings of discourses and events (Martin 1996: 106–12). As in the quote below, at times in *Volatile Bodies* Grosz also positions the biological as more fixed than the social (the biological is theorised as a limit on the social rather than the other way around). This emphasis allows an active/passive split to resurface as biology is positioned as a passive limitation on the social:

The body is constrained by its biological limits – limits, incidentally, whose framework or 'stretchability' we cannot yet know, we cannot presume, even if we must presume some limits. The body is not open to all the whims, wishes, and hopes of the subject: the human body, for example, cannot fly in the air, it cannot breathe underwater unaided by prostheses, it requires a broad range of temperatures and environmental supports, without which it risks collapse and death.

(Grosz 1994: 187)

In his review article, Pheng Cheah argues that the radicality of both Grosz's and Butler's theorising of the body is undercut by the positioning of materiality as negative constraint (Cheah 1996). In Cheah's reading,

Grosz's reliance on the Lacanian notion of 'the natural lack in mankind', and Butler's focus on the performative role of language and signification, mean that they focus only on humans as active and view non-human nature as passive. In relation to Grosz, for example, Cheah writes:

> [D]espite her astute observation that the body is indeterminably positioned between material weightiness and cultural variability so that either trait may be used depending on whether one opposes essentialism or social constructionism, the emphasis on strategic use favours variability as a higher level of strategic cognition. Often the weightiness of matter or nature in general is played down. Or inhuman nature carries an unfavourable connotation in comparison with human nature which is fluid and capable of retranscription.
>
> *(Cheah 1996: 127)*

In her more recent book, *Time Travels*, Grosz (2005) places more emphasis on the biological (what she calls 'nature'), deliberately privileging the analysis of the subordinate term in the nature/culture binary. She theorises nature as an active force, one that enables rather than limits culture: 'I am interested in the ways in which nature, composed of the biological and the material, organic and inorganic systems that sustain life, incites and produces culture, that is, the ways in which the biological enables rather than limits and directs social and cultural life' (Grosz 2005: 43).[11] This change in emphasis potentially provides a more positive role for biological actors such as hormones. Grosz claims that 'sexual difference, the systematically differing morphologies of (most) living bodies, operates not only at the level of the body-as-a-whole, but also within the body's microscopic functions and processes' (Grosz 2005: 195). Despite the use of the word 'microscopic', Grosz does not analyse entities such as hormones, cells or genes, writing instead of 'messy biology' in an abstract, philosophical sense.[12] Remaining in the realm of such abstraction, Grosz is unable to address the ways in which 'nature' is produced through contemporary technoscientific practices.

---

[11] In this work, Grosz specifically distances herself from Butler, arguing that Butler understands subjectivity as based on human interaction and fails to take into account the activity of the non-human (or 'inhuman') world (Grosz 2005: 189–190; see also 78–9). Whilst I agree that Butler focuses her attention on human actions, I consider Grosz's assessment of Butler's work that 'what slips out, what disappears, is stuff, the real, biology, nature, matter' harsh (Grosz 2005: 78). As discussed in the Introduction, Butler explicitly refers to non-human actors such as hormones and, particularly in her most recent book *Undoing Gender*, highlights questions of materiality and (human) biological existence (see, for example, 2004: 31, 226).

[12] The one scientific body of work addressed in any detail by Grosz is that of Charles Darwin.

Despite this limitation, Grosz's theorisation of the interimplication of nature and culture moves us away from questioning whether the body is social or biological towards asking how an examination of the body demonstrates the limitations of these categories. In relation to the sciences discussed above, this approach radically undermines the assumption that complex processes can be divided into entities that are either biologically or socially caused. The problematisation of the biological/social distinction produced by feminist theories of the body means that questions about the causes of sexed behaviours must be fundamentally reframed.

Popular science

[B]odies as objects of knowledge are material-semiotic generative nodes. Their *boundaries* materialize in social interaction. Boundaries are drawn by mapping practices; 'objects' do not preexist as such. Objects are boundary projects. But boundaries shift from within; boundaries are very tricky. What boundaries provisionally contain remains generative, productive of meanings and bodies. Siting (sighting) boundaries is a risky practice.

(Haraway 1991: 200–1)

In contrast to Grosz, Haraway emphasises the ways in which bodies are produced through technoscientific and other practices, describing such practices as 'social interaction'. In her terms, technoscientific affirmations of the social/biological distinction in describing bodies in sexually differentiated forms are a boundary-making exercise, a material-discursive practice that allows scientists to make claims about the world that have significant effects on the lives of humans and non-humans and their environments. Like Grosz and other feminist theorists, she argues that the binary oppositions structuring western thought set up particular ways in which certain more powerfully positioned humans can relate to other less powerfully situated humans, to non-humans and to the world. This relation is one of domination and is replicated in the hierarchised nature of the binary itself, where the dominant term (the social, mind, man) 'orders the silent term [biology, body, woman] by a logic of appropriation' (Haraway 1991: 250, n. 10). Such claims about the world are facilitated by the popularisation of technoscientific discourses in popular books and magazines.

Psychological and behavioural neuroendocrinological theories tend to lean towards biologistic explanations of the role of sex hormones in the production of behaviours and psychologies. This tendency is vastly increased in texts (books, magazine articles, television documentaries, websites) representing these sciences for a popular audience. In these representations, biology in the form of hormones is seen to be directly and simply responsible for all kinds of sexual differences.

In her analysis of North American media, Dorothy Nelkin shows that coverage of science rarely includes theoretical work. Most reports of science are about 'facts'. 'A notable exception', however, 'are those theories of behavior that bear on controversial social stereotypes' (Nelkin 1987: 27). Thus theories regarding human differences such as evolutionary theories, biological determinism and sociobiology have received an unusual amount of attention, with stories about sex differences being the most common. In relation to sociobiology in particular, Nelkin argues that 'In selecting this subject for extensive coverage, journalists are in effect using a controversial theory to legitimize a particular point of view' (Nelkin 1987: 27). Her analysis of media reports of sociobiology finds that the scientific controversies around such work are often not reported and the claims that such sciences make are presented as definitive facts.

Articles in *Time* magazine and *The Atlantic Monthly*, for example, discuss the importance of sex hormones in the production of sexual difference and homosexuality (Gorman 1992; Burr 1993). In both these articles, the role of biology in the production of sexual and sexuality differences is promoted as an antidote to the perceived exaggeration of social influences. The subheading in the *Time* article reads, 'Scientists are discovering that gender differences have as much to do with the biology of the brain as with the way we are raised' (Gorman 1992: 30). The story told here is that the role of biology has been repressed as politically incorrect, but 'Now that it is O.K. to admit the possibility, the search for sexual differences has expanded into nearly every branch of the life sciences' (Gorman 1992: 32). This view of the history of scientific research into this area is blatantly incorrect as such a search has been steadily under way for at least two centuries. This view, however, allows the author to present biological arguments as the ignored part of the nature/nurture equation.

Articles such as these often downplay the minimal and problematic nature of the evidence cited: 'What is striking about many of the articles on sociobiology', Nelkin found, 'is how easily reporters slide from noting a provocative theory to citing it as fact, even when they know the supporting evidence may be flimsy' (Nelkin 1987: 30). Chandler Burr's article in *The Atlantic* (1993), for example, strongly affirms the likelihood that homosexuality will in the future be found to be biologically based. Although reference is made to 'the web of complexities', Burr argues that 'it is becoming clearer that biological factors play a role in determining human sexual orientation', quoting two scientists who state that in their lifetime a biological explanation for homosexuality will be found (Burr 1993: 65). Like the science they report, articles like these pretend to have accounted for the complexities wrought by the social but still to have found that the biological is more important.

Other media representations are more directly biologically determinist, although in their titles and general tone there is a sense of irony that undercuts a strictly adherent or naïve reading. An article in the *Sydney Morning Herald* reprinted from *The New York Times* and entitled 'Sex on the brain – it depends on the gender' provides an example. This article reports that men and women experience connections between sexual arousal and desire differently, and that this difference 'shows up in the brain' (O'Connor 2004: 7). Similarly, a piece in *The Guardian* entitled 'Finger points to good research skills' suggests that men's and women's different aptitudes for professions is determined by prenatal hormones, as indicated by the relative lengths of the second and fourth fingers (Curtis 2004). Exposure to more oestrogen in the womb is 'genetically linked' to a longer index finger, whilst testosterone exposure is linked to a longer ring finger. The research described studied the finger lengths of various scientists and, according to journalist Polly Curtis, demonstrates that 'male scientists are good at research because they have the same hormone levels as women'. There is no mention here of social explanations of why women and men might excel in different types of work, but the generally humorous tone – which lightly mocks male scientists for being like women – turns the piece into a form of social commentary rather than a serious intervention into the contemporary politics of the gendered workplace.

Other less humorous popular representations violently reject *any* emphasis on the social. One notable example is the book *Brain Sex: The Real Difference Between Men and Women*, by Anne Moir and David Jessel, which was made into a successful television documentary series of the same name. In their introduction, Moir and Jessel state their basic position: that scientific research has proved beyond any rational doubt that sexual differences in bodies and behaviours are biological and caused by hormones' effect on the brain. 'Men are different from women', the first sentence proclaims: 'The sexes are different because their brains are different' (Moir and Jessel 1991: 5). *Brain Sex* positions itself as a rejection of the foolish desires of the 'apostles of sexual sameness' who claim that sexual differences in behaviours and aptitudes are socially constructed (Moir and Jessel 1991: 128) and suggests that at last the time has come for the truth to come out:

> Until recently, behavioural differences between the sexes have been explained
> away by social conditioning ... Scant attention was paid to the biological view
> that we may be what we are because of the way we are made. Today, there is too
> much evidence for the sociological argument to prevail. The argument of
> biology at last provides a comprehensive, and scientifically provable framework
> within which we can begin to understand why we are who we are.
>
> *(Moir and Jessel 1991: 5–6)*

The biological explanation Moir and Jessel report is very simple: the
brain is affected by hormones in the womb which make it male or female,
and then later in puberty this 'pre-wired' brain (Moir and Jessel 1991: 6) is
encouraged even more firmly to be male or female: 'That is, female
hormones have a much stronger impact upon a brain which is, by its
very design, more sensitive to their effect, while a male brain is predis-
posed, again by design, to react to male hormone' (Moir and Jessel 1991:
70). With this simple formula, gained from reading and citing the research
analysed above, Moir and Jessel go on to explain a range of phenomena
that are demonstrated to be caused by hormones: boys' and girls' different
performances on school tests; men's and women's different responses to
babies (including who does the work of looking after them); male and
female experiences of sexuality (including men's promiscuity and women's
frigidity); social class; and the different occupations and pay rates of men
and women. Moir and Jessel argue that these 'natural' and hormonally
caused conditions are impossible to successfully change, and indeed,
should probably not be changed. As they claim in their introduction, the
explanations they give of sexual difference seem 'plausible' (Moir and
Jessel 1991: 6) and reassuring. 'Better, too, to welcome and exploit the
complementary differences between men and women', the book argues, as
this is sure to 'make us happier' (Moir and Jessel 1991: 7). Readers could
easily go away from this book convinced that the world is basically all right
and will be even better when we stop trying to create equality between men
and women.

Popular books such as these, which use the authority and perceived
neutrality of the science they report to make deeply political claims, are
clearly dangerous. The long list of scientists thanked in the acknowledge-
ments who 'patiently answered questions and/or sent their latest research'
(Moir and Jessel 1991: 1) suggests that this type of writing may be a
sanctioned part of the scientific enterprise that allows more virulent and
political claims to be made to a different (and presumably less scientifically
literate) audience. This suggestion is supported by Nelkin's finding that
scientists often encouraged wide-ranging interpretations of their work in

media interviews – interpretations that are not to be found in their more careful publications in scientific journals (Nelkin 1987).

Moir's and Jessel's book is also exemplary in the stunning ignorance and sarcastic aggression with which all social science and feminist arguments about the cultural construction of sexual difference and sexual inequalities are discussed and rejected. Such arguments are presented as the views of extremists whose true desire is to destroy the 'natural' differences between men and women. The opinions of those stressing social factors are referred to as 'dismissive, politically motivated, [and] fashionable' (Moir and Jessel 1991: 19) and the theorists themselves are presented as 'the legions of social engineers who impatiently await' the newborn baby in order to construct a sexually neutral child (Moir and Jessel 1991: 20). Moir and Jessel simply do not pay any serious attention to arguments stressing non-biological factors in human development. The conclusion of *Brain Sex* is that 'the argument about the existence of brain sex differences has been won' (Moir and Jessel 1991: 179). 'It now seems a little strange that the battle ever had to be fought at all, when men and women are so obviously different in physique and behaviour', Moir and Jessel write as their book completes its circle (Moir and Jessel 1991: 179). All we have learnt is that what was already obvious through simple observation is true and that the status quo should be maintained for nature's sake.

Simon Baron-Cohen ends *The Essential Difference* in a similar vein, stating that 'a central tenet of this book is that the male and female brain differ from each other, but that *overall* one is not better or worse than the other' (Baron-Cohen 2004: 184, emphasis in original). Claiming that the 'society at present is likely to be biased towards accepting the extreme female brain and stigmatizes the extreme male brain', however, he adds a different twist. Positioning men as needing to experience 'a resurgence of pride at the things they do well', his 'hope', he adds, 'is that the stigmatizing [that men currently suffer] will soon be history' (Baron-Cohen 2004: 185). Baron-Cohen thus positions his book as a counter-attack on 'some [unnamed] authors' who 'want to oppress men' in their rejection of biologically essentialist theories of sex differences (Baron-Cohen, 2004: 11).[13]

---

[13] Baron-Cohen's argument is so extraordinary it is worth quoting in more detail. In a chapter subsection entitled 'The politics of studying sex differences', he espouses a commitment to reducing inequality in society and writes, 'Discussing sex differences of course drops you straight into the heart of the political correctness debate. Some people say that even looking for sex differences reveals a sexist mind that is looking for ways to perpetuate the historical inequalities women have suffered. There is no doubt at all about the reality of

A feminist response: rejecting essentialism?

The mainstream sciences describing the role of hormones in the production of sexually differentiated behaviours tend towards biologistic explanations. This is achieved through the devaluing and reduction of social explanations, caused in part by adherence to a social/biological dichotomy. Despite the existence of other technoscientific knowledge challenging these biologistic models, these explanations are routinely used, particularly in popular scientific literature and media reports, to justify and affirm oppressive situations and institutions. They do also, however – as described by historians Stephanie Kenen (1997) and Jennifer Terry (1997) – have a long history of being used to advocate tolerance of differences. In either case, these theories are always political.

One major feminist response to such biologistic explanations has been to reject them as essentialist. Grosz defines essentialism as 'the attribution of a fixed essence to women' and defines biologism as 'a particular form of essentialism in which women's essence is defined in terms of their biological capacities' (Grosz 1990: 334). The problems of essentialist claims are listed by Grosz: '[T]hey are necessarily ahistorical; they confuse social relations with fixed attributes; they see these fixed attributes as inherent limitations to social change; and they refuse to take seriously the historical and geographical differences between women – differences between women across different cultures as well as within a single culture' (Grosz 1990: 335). Work such as that produced by Reinisch and colleagues and Baron-Cohen meets this definition (indeed, Baron-Cohen chooses the word 'essential' to describe the biological differences he studies).

the oppression of women, and the last thing I want to do is to perpetuate this. Nor for that matter do I want to oppress men, which has been the aim of some authors. Questions about sex differences can still be asked without aiming to oppress either sex' (Baron-Cohen 2004: 11). Baron-Cohen goes on to claim that he had to postpone finishing his book in the 1990s because 'the topic was just too politically sensitive', but that his friends (including women and some feminists) later convinced him that 'the time is ripe for such a discussion' (Baron-Cohen 2004: 11). Many feminists today, he states, rather than 'assert[ing] that there was nothing that men could do that a woman could not do equally well . . . have become rather proud that there are things that most women can do that most men cannot do as well' (Baron-Cohen 2004: 12). In terms of engaging with social explanations of sex differences, Baron-Cohen is less sarcastic than Moir and Jessel, but he repeatedly asserts that social explanations are unconvincing in relation to children less than four years old; that very young children have not had enough time to learn social conventions or are unable to articulate or recognise social gender norms (Baron-Cohen 2004: 86–95). In this chapter on culture, Baron-Cohen fails to engage with any social-scientific or feminist work on gender and like the other scientists discussed above, utilises an extremely narrow understanding of what 'culture' is and how it might shape children's behaviour.

However, the essentialism debates of the 1980s and 1990s have led many feminists to question the value of critiques that stop at the accusation of essentialism. This questioning has centred on issues concerning bodily differences between the sexes, asking, for example: If we critique biologistic explanations of sexual differences, what happens to the body, or to bodily differences? Do we have to reject all descriptions of biology in rejecting essentialism? Or can there be some other way of theorising biology that does not posit it as either primary or unchanging?[14]

For some theorists, the idea that essentialism cannot be simply rejected is based on the belief that feminism needs to retain some notion of 'women' to survive as a political movement. They argue that feminism must retain this word, even at the expense of opening itself up to the accusation of essentialising and thus not properly accounting for differences between women, and/or claiming some sort of defining meaning of 'women' that does not exist. Braidotti puts it strongly: '[A] feminist woman theoretician who is interested in thinking about sexual difference and the feminine today cannot afford not to be essentialist' (Braidotti 1989: 93).

When feminist theorists take this stand for what Gayatri Spivak names a 'strategic' use of essentialism (Spivak with Grosz 1984: 11), however, they very rarely base their strategic use of the word 'women' on a biological definition. Instead they tend to rely on some sort of shared cultural oppression, or lived and/or psychical embodiment. In *Volatile Bodies*, for example, Grosz stresses a notion of sexual difference that is related to a shared experience of embodiment. She claims that some experiences of the cultural, political, signified and signifying body are, in general if not in their specifics, shared by women: the experiences of menstruation and lactation. Grosz is quick to point out that:

> This irreducible specificity in no way universalizes the particular ways in which women experience their bodies and bodily flows. But given the social significance of these bodily processes that are invested in and by the processes of reproduction, all women's bodies are marked as different to men's (and inferior to them) particularly at those bodily regions where women's differences are most visibly manifest.
>
> *(Grosz 1994: 207)*

---

[14] This kind of questioning has lead in some cases to reevaluations of technoscientific knowledges and to feminist work that mines technoscience for intellectual resources for thinking differently about the relationships between biologies, bodies and worlds (see, for example, Hird 2004; Wilson 2005). This feminist work is part of a broader change in social scientific and humanities-based approaches to technoscience. For a critical discussion of this change, see Roberts and Mackenzie 2006.

Thus she relies on a notion of a certain commonality of women's bodily
experiences while at the same time refusing to name this body 'biological'.
In a footnote she explains further: 'I am not advocating a naturalist or even
a universalist attribute. Nonetheless, it is also true that all women, whatever the details of their physiology and fertility, are culturally understood
in terms of these bodily flows' (Grosz 1994: 228).

The distinction between the biological and the morphological body is
central to Grosz's argument. On the question of the relation of the biological body to essentialism, Gayatri Spivak makes an important point in
an interview with Ellen Rooney, who asks if our confusion about how to
theorise the body is the root of the problem of essentialism. Interestingly,
Rooney follows this question with a reference to a newspaper article that
stated that women find it hard to find their cars during menstruation
because of hormonal changes. Spivak interrupts and says 'Really?
I didn't see that. It gives me an answer to the question' (Spivak, with
Rooney 1994: 176). By this, she presumably means that the answer to
Rooney's question about the central role of the biological body is 'yes'.
Rooney then goes on to ask Spivak about her attempts to address bodies,
and Spivak replies:

> I am against universalizing in that way. I mean I would look at why they're
> essentializing, rather than to say 'this is bad' necessarily, because I think there is
> something, some biological remnant in the notion of gender, even in the good
> notion of gender. Biology doesn't just disappear, except it should not be offered
> as a ground of all explanations. So basically on that, you know, I'm a non
> foundationalist in that sense especially when grounds are found to justify bad
> politics. So it's almost as if I'm going at it the other way, a sort of deductive anti-
> essentialist, how is the essence being used?
>
> *(Spivak 1994: 176–7)*

Spivak thus rejects an outright refusal of the notion of biology and
focusses instead on an examination of how biology is used to make certain
political claims. She stresses that there is no biology (or way of thinking
about bodies and their functions) that is somehow pure, untainted by
culture or the social: there is, for her, no 'body as such' that can be thought
outside of cultural systems of thought. In this her position comes close to
that of Grosz. She states:

> But apart from that I would say that biology, a biology, is one way of thinking
> the systematicity of the body. The body, like all other things, cannot be thought
> as such. Like all other things I have never tried to approach the body as such.
> I do take the extreme ecological view that the body as such has no possible
> outline ... You know, if one really thinks of the body as such, there is no

possible outline of the body as such ... There are thinkings of the systematicity
of the body, there are value codings of the body. The body, as such, cannot
be thought, and I certainly cannot approach it.

(Spivak 1994: 177)

Spivak's position on essentialism and the body is useful here. It avoids
simplistic rejections of scientific arguments as essentialist (they are essentialist and therefore bad) and instead argues for an examination of the
political uses of essentialist claims. Also, her position on biology avoids
the reaffirmation of the biology/social distinction by refusing an absolute
denial of the role of biology. We can assume that some sort of biological
exists, but it cannot be thought outside of discourse.

The danger to feminist criticisms of scientific positions such as those
describing the role of hormones in producing sex differences is that if
biology is simply rejected as essentialist, simplistic, or just plain unbearable, it is reinstated as unknowable and beyond the social, beyond feminism (see also Grosz 1999: 31–2; Wilson 1999). In turn, giving biology this
status means that the social/biological distinction is affirmed rather than
deconstructed. Equally pertinent are scientific findings discussed above
that even the behaviour of supposedly 'simple' animals such as rats and
chickens cannot be explained as simply biological (or non-social).
Chapter 2, similarly, showed that basic endocrinological physiology is
unable to sustain an argument that the sexed body itself is 'simply biological'. Instead there are many complicated interactions and congruences
that fluctuate and combine to produce any particular sexed body at any
particular moment. Feminist theory, then, does itself a disservice by pre-
suming that biology is the opposite of the social, or that the distinction
between the social and the biological is anywhere clear or knowable. For it
seems always that one is inside the other already: the social in the biological
and, perhaps more perturbingly for feminist theory, the biological in the
social. Neither can be understood in separation from the other. As Spivak
says, 'the body, like all other things cannot be thought as such' (Spivak
1994: 177).

Sex hormones play varied roles in the production of sex differences
across different discourses. These range from simple determination of
differences via gonads, through the structuring of brains and mysterious
'predispositions', to a more complex view of co-action with the social
environment. Whilst feminist theorists have successfully argued that the
biological cannot be directly approached, we need effective ways of thinking through these historically powerful roles. To focus on the co-construction
or 'interimplication' of the biological and the social, rather than replicating

their division, provides an alternative approach to technoscientific narratives of hormones and sex.

Narrating hormones and sex: two illustrative examples

In her recent book, *The Companion Species Manifesto*, Haraway uses the term 'naturecultures' to talk about the interimplication of the biological and the social. In describing the historically specific naturecultures of dogs, she writes,

> Dogs are about the inescapable, contradictory story of relationships –
> co-constitutive relationships in which none of the partners pre-exist the relating,
> and the relating is never done once and for all. Historical specificity and
> contingent mutability rule all the way down, into nature and culture, into
> naturecultures. There is no foundation; there are only elephants supporting
> elephants all the way down.
>
> *(Haraway 2003: 12)*

This understanding of the naturecultures of dogs is brought to life in a description of sexual play between Haraway's spayed female dog, Cayenne Pepper and her 'intact' canine friend, Willem. 'Willem', Haraway writes,

> is a randy, gentle utterly inexperienced, adolescent male soul. Cayenne does not
> have an estrus hormone in her body (but let us not forget those very much
> present adrenal cortices pumping out so-called androgens that get lots of the
> credit for juicing up mammalian desire in males and females). She is, however,
> one turned on little bitch with Willem, and he is INTERESTED. She does not do
> this with any other dog, 'intact' or not. None of their sexual play has anything to
> do with remotely functional heterosexual mating behavior – no efforts of
> Willem to mount, no presenting of an attractive female backside, not much
> genital sniffing, no whining and pacing, none of all that reproductive stuff. No,
> here we have pure polymorphous perversity that is so dear to the hearts of all
> of us who came of age in the 1960s reading Norman O. Brown.
>
> *(Haraway 2003: 99, emphasis in original)*

In this description, Haraway refuses to describe the dogs' activities as reproductive (they are clearly not) and (seriously) jokes with her readers that these pleasure-oriented canine erotics can be compared to modern American human sexual practices: Willem, she writes, is 'what feminists of my generation would call a considerate lover' (Haraway 2003: 100). What is most interesting here to me, however, is Haraway's reference to hormones. Whilst she is describing Cayenne Pepper and Willem's activities as particular to their relationship and as pleasure-, rather than reproduction-oriented, she also mentions 'biology' in a way that neither denies its role nor gives it causal credit. Hormones are described both as substances that get 'pumped out' of 'cortices' but also as entities historically positioned in narratives: she refers to 'so-called androgens' (to note, presumably, that such hormones were thought to belong to males only) and states that these hormones 'get lots of the credit for juicing up desire' in mammals. This clever and funny piece of writing enacts hormones as naturecultures: hormones are material-semiotic actors, always both at the same time. 'Flesh and signifier, bodies and words, stories and words: these are joined in naturecultures', Haraway (2003: 20) writes. This is why stories are central to studying technoscience: there can be no reference to biology (to something like hormones) that is not a story, connected to other stories. Thus the role of the science-studies scholar, in Haraway's view, is to examine and retell the stories of technoscience: 'Inverting meanings; transposing the body of communication; remolding, remodelling; swervings that tell the truth: I tell stories about stories all the way down' (Haraway 2003: 20–1).

Haraway's storytelling about her dogs contrasts starkly to other, less challenging, hormonal stories. Family therapist Steve Biddulph's popular how-to book, *Raising Boys*, for example, suggests that boys provoke particular parenting challenges because of their exposure to testosterone (*in utero*, at four years of age and at puberty). This exposure, Biddulph states, causes the average boy to have 30 per cent more muscle bulk than the average girl (he does not mention at what age). In turn, this extra bulk means that 'boys are stronger and their bodies are more inclined to action' (Biddulph 1997: 33). He then asserts that boys 'even have more red blood cells (the original red-blooded boy!)'. From this, Biddulph extrapolates that 'we have to give boys plenty of chance to exercise' and that 'boys will need extra help to control themselves from hitting each other and girls' (Biddulph 1997: 33). What is notable here is the way that Biddulph moves from a statement of 'fact' to a metaphor (from red blood cells to red-blooded) and then presents gendered behaviour differences (boys are more likely than girls to hit others) as something stemming directly from the biological fact (when really it stems only from his metaphor). Logically, boys having more red blood cells could only have an indirect relation to how often they hit others – for Biddulph, this is a direct step (although one he can only make through a jokey metaphor).

In developing his hormonal sex story further, Biddulph cites evidence from horses, rats and monkeys, arguing that testosterone 'causes energetic and boisterous behaviour' (Biddulph 1997: 39). 'The point', Biddulph asserts, 'is that testosterone influences the brain and makes boys more concerned with rank and competition' (Biddulph 1997: 40). This point is derived from a direct comparison between boys and the social behaviour of adult monkeys. In order to shore up this rather stretched comparison, Biddulph moves on to human evolution, making reference to the specific demands made on men's bodies in hunter-gatherer societies: 'Men's bodies were better at rapid bursts of strength but more likely to be laid low by a dose of 'flu or an ingrown toenail!' he writes. The differences between women's gathering and men's hunting tasks, he argues, gradually meant that 'we ended up with a species with slight but significant differences between male and female bodies and brains'. These differences continue today, Biddulph suggests, in third world countries where 'men often do not work as hard as the women. Presumably', he adds, eschewing any reference to social hierarchies, 'they are waiting to fight someone or hunt something!' (Biddulph 1997: 43). To end his chapter, Biddulph summarises: 'Some girls have a lot of testosterone but, on the whole, it's a boy thing – and needs our understanding, not blame or ridicule. Testosterone equals vitality, and it's our job to honour it and steer it in healthy directions' (Biddulph 1997: 47). The remainder of the book teaches parents (mostly men) how to do this job.[15]

Biddulph's book is in stark contrast to Haraway's manifesto in several illustrative respects. Firstly, he consistently attempts to isolate hormones as causal agents in human behaviour; his stories reduce testosterone to something very simple ('vitality') that should be 'honored'. Like Haraway, Biddulph tells stories about sex and behaviour, but these stories refuse to acknowledge the historical or cultural contingency of their foundations. Stories are built upon one another – children on ancient humans on animals – but these are seen as stacks of inevitable truths, not as the partial connections of contingent histories. Like Haraway, Biddulph's stories mix up biochemicals, people, animals, values and stories in unsettling ways, but do so in order to narrate a truth that claims to be straightforward, apolitical and clear (and one that promotes the interests of boys and men).

---

[15] Like Baron-Cohen and Moir and Jessel, Biddulph sets his argument against 'the fashionable theory for the last thirty years ... that boys and girls have no differences other than those that we give them through conditioning' (Biddulph 1997: 31). Holders of these ideas are described as 'fanatical' and as responsible for creating an atmosphere in which 'research into gender differences became a taboo subject, because nobody wanted to be seen to be setting back the cause of women's liberation'. In a familiar logic, Biddulph then argues that 'nowadays ... there is a willingness to see that some differences do exist which are not socially created, and that these differences are okay' (Biddulph 1997: 32).

Messaging as multidirectional flow

Haraway describes her understanding of the interimplication of the bio-logical and the social in terms of kinship networks and 'multidirectional flows'. Using a gardening metaphor, she writes:

> Like the productions of a decadent gardener who can't keep good distinctions between natures and cultures straight, the shape of my kin networks looks more like a trellis or an esplanade than a tree. You can't tell up from down, and every thing seems to go sideways. Such snake-like, sidewinding traffic is one of my themes. My garden is full of snakes, full of trellises, full of indirection. Instructed by evolutionary population biologists and bioanthropologists, I know that multidirectional gene flow – multidirectional flows of bodies and values – is and has always been the name of the game of life on earth.
>
> *(Haraway 2003: 9)*

This description of the 'multidirectional flows of bodies and values' also articulates the messaging actions of hormones. The analysis of scientific and popular texts undertaken in this chapter has demonstrated that tech-noscientific explanations of the role of sex hormones in producing sexed behaviours always 'go sideways' in order to make their arguments. They consistently rely on social norms of sex/gender and reproductive hetero-sexuality in order to make arguments about the 'natural' connections between hormones and sexual behaviours. For feminists, these are the potentially poisonous snakes in the gardens of biological psychology and neuroendocrinology.

Although this chapter has been critical in its approach to these sciences, I want to suggest, as I did in Chapter 2, that this analysis is ultimately positive. The sideways connections repeatedly made in these technoscien-tific fields point to spaces in which the interimplication of the social and the biological might be acknowledged and explored. Rather than determining factors, hormones could be refigured in these discourses as active messag-ing agents, about which new stories can be told: stories that neither deny hormones' activities nor afford them narrow roles. Part III takes this suggestion forward into the realms of contemporary biomedicine. Working with the examples of hormone-replacement therapies and endocrine-disrupting chemicals, I experiment with theorising hormones as active messengers to see what differences this might make to how hormones, bodies and health are articulated in contemporary western cultures.

PART III

Hormone cultures

4

Elixirs of sex: hormone-replacement therapies and contemporary life

Internationally, millions of women take sex hormones in the form of pharmaceuticals to address a range of conditions: unwanted fertility, menstrual problems, infertility and menopausal symptoms. This extensive consumption of hormones takes place at a time in which taking multiple drugs 'for life' is a widely accepted practice; a mode of life promoted strongly in the United States where pharmaceutical products are advertised on television, radio and magazines (Dumit 2002, 2005).[1] Particularly as hormone-replacement treatments for menopausal women, hormones constitute a highly profitable business: in 2001, for example, one brand of hormone-replacement therapy (HRT) was the best-selling drug on the global market, making US$2 billion profit for its manufacturer, Wyeth (Seaman 2003: 106; Morrison 2004). Named Premarin[TM] after its source, this drug is made from urine collected from 40,000 pregnant mares controversially stabled for this purpose. Debates about the provenance of this drug are entered into by animal rights campaigners with much intensity, foregrounding links between women and female animals; between human and non-human animal reproductivity. These debates also highlight the surprising economic and symbolic flows through which hormones gain and confer biovalue (Waldby 2000).[2]

---

[1] Dumit (2005: 11) describes this as 'dependent normality', a bio-social condition in which 'being diagnosed and dependent on medication is rendered ordinary'.

[2] All other brands of HRT are synthetically manufactured. Animal welfare campaigners are working to halt this use of horses, which, they argue, results in the extensive slaughter and selling for food of unwanted foals removed earlier than usual from their mothers (see, for example, www.horseofct.org/premarin.htm. Last accessed 25 September 2006). The theme of connections between human and non-human animals in hormone circuits is developed in Chapter 6.

This chapter theorises the exogenous hormones of HRT as messengers of sex. It asks how taking HRT came to be an accepted part of life for millions of menopausal women in the wealthy west whilst remaining unavailable for many women living in other parts of the world. It also examines the history and current status of HRT for men, asking whether the contemporary push to persuade men to take HRT signals a significant change in the production of sexed bodies and sex/gender relations. Investigating historical and con-temporary HRT discourses, I discuss the significance of sexed embodiment to contemporary bio-social conceptions of healthy existence. How are sex/gender differences connected to life – and opposed to death – in HRT discourses? As an 'elixir of life' is HRT also an elixir of sex? Thinking about forms of HRT as ways in which hormones message sex, I argue that practices and discourses built around moving exogenous sex hormones into women and men (re)produce particular embodiments, materialising histor-ically specific configurations of sex, race and class.

Menopause for women and men

In 1966, HRT guru Robert A. Wilson suggested in his popular book *Feminine Forever* that menopause affected men via their relationships to symptomatic women. 'The menopause covers such a wide range of physi-cal and emotional symptoms', he wrote, 'that the implications are by no means confined to the woman. Her husband, her family, and her entire relationship to the outside world are affected almost as strongly as her own body.' The benefits of HRT, or 'hormonal cure' as Wilson called it, could only 'be properly appreciated' in this 'broader context' (Wilson 1966: 80). Menopausal women's subjectivities and bodies are understood in this influential work as pathologically overflowing boundaries of contained selfhood. Such overflow, Wilson (1966: 18) suggests, should be 'cured' or 'prevented' by long-term hormonal medication.

Today, the effects of menopause on men are more direct, as 'the average man' now suffers from menopause himself and thus also requires hormo-nal therapy. Speaking of HRT for men in his popular book, *The Testosterone Syndrome*, would-be guru Eugene Shippen asserts:

> Resistance will fade. Testosterone therapy has every prospect of becoming for men what estrogen therapy is now for millions of women. The male meno-pause, a real tragedy in the midlife of the average man, has had its day. I am going to put a stake through its ugly little heart.
>
> *(Shippen and Fryer 1998: ix)*

Like Wilson's description of menopausal women, Shippen's characterisation of aging men depends on a model of aging as pathology (and youth as normative) and of sex/gender as a static and fixed entity that must be maintained, even at high cost. His vampiric analogy conveys a strong sense of disgust regarding aging; the loss of masculinity associated with decline in testosterone levels is figured as inhuman and evil, something – reminiscent of de Beauvoir's female body – to be struggled against and even eventually killed.

Within mainstream medical literature, this creature with the 'ugly little heart' is defined as 'a syndrome in aging men consist[ing] of physical, sexual, and psychologic symptoms that include weakness, fatigue, reduced muscle and bone mass, impaired hematopoesis, oligiospermia, sexual dysfunction, depression, anxiety, irritability, insomnia, memory impairment, and reduced cognitive function' (Lund *et al.* 1999: 951). The male menopause or andropause – described more simply as 'a complex of symptoms in aging men who have low testosterone levels' (Bain 2001: 91) – recently provoked the question, 'Is it time for the geriatrician to treat it?' (Morely 2001: 263). Over the last five years, research has gradually established that testosterone levels do decline in at least a significant proportion of men as they age. In an editorial in the *Journal of Gerontology*, geriatrician John E. Morely states that '70 per cent of males aged 70 years are hypogonadal', or in other words, produce such low levels of testosterone as to become 'symptomatic' (Morely 2001: 263). Clinical trials of hormone-replacement therapies for these men have shown that testosterone can have some impact on 'reversing' andropausal symptoms. Morely concludes 'the emerging data seem to create a clear imperative for the geriatrician to look aggressively for hypogonadism in the older man and treat it when it is present' (Morely 2001: 265).

The 'aggressive' search for andropause and hormonal treatments for it borrow deliberately from the more familiar scenario of hormone-replacement therapy for women. The experience and treatment of menopause is mentioned in most medical, scientific and popular articles on the andropause. The understanding of aging processes as treatable deficiency diseases is significant in both cases, as are certain 'delivery systems' such as patches and pills. More insidiously, potential connections between taking hormones and increased risks of cancer are also shared.

Economic incentives for the development of HRT for women and men are powerful. As aging specialist John B. McKinlay remarks, 'There is a very strong interest in treating aging men for profit, just as there is for menopausal women' (McKinlay, in Hoberman and Yesalis 1995: 65).

Commenting in *Clinical Endocrinology*, Eberhard Nieschlag similarly suggests, 'If ongoing studies succeed in documenting the benefits of testosterone replacement therapy in male senescence – without negative effects on the prostate – the market would grow enormously ... If this dream of the pharmaceutical companies is to come true, another gap between men and women would be closed, since HRT is already standard therapy in menopausal women' (Nieschlag 1996: 261). In the context of contemporary bio-socialities in which taking drugs 'for life' is normative, this dream of closing a gap between traditional and new users of HRT arguably has real potential. This dream is also bolstered by the aging of western populations, which provides a constantly increasing market for such medications.

HRT histories

Whilst the twenty-first-century dream of providing testosterone-based hormone therapy for men is in one sense 'barely 10 years old' (Bain 2001: 91), it has long been part of sex endocrinology. Historically, endocrinological research has been closely tied with the production of hormones as medical products and specifically as anti-aging medications designed to promote, amongst other things, the maintenance of sexual drive. The foundational story of sex endocrinology – that of Charles Brown-Séquard's injections of crushed dog's testicles – revolves around this dream of using hormones to renew the youth (and in particular the youthful sexual drive) of aging men. After an initial burst of work on men, however, HRT research quite quickly became almost exclusively focused on women, remaining so for the last fifty years.

How did HRT come to be a medication for women? Why did an industry develop around supplying hormones to women, rather than men, for this purpose? In her history of sex endocrinology, Nelly Oudshoorn gives a practical answer. She argues that research materials were available for research on hormones for women but were unavailable for research on men. Correlates of the institutions surrounding women's reproductive systems simply did not exist for men. Using social network theory, Oudshoorn argues that existing actors in women's health could take up and use hormones, thus establishing a network, whilst around men's health these actors were missing (Oudshoorn 1994: 82–111; 1996a: 125–6).

As described in Chapter 1, endocrinologists succeeded in isolating oestrogen in 1929 and testosterone in 1931. This began an energetic industry in producing these hormones both for research and for medical products. In order to obtain pure extracts of sex hormones, tons of raw materials such as ovaries, placentae and testes were required and laboratories made arrangements with slaughterhouses for supplies. Another source of sex hormones was human urine. Oudshoorn points out that gynaecological clinics could easily obtain samples from their pregnant patients, so research materials for work on ovarian hormones were 'both abundant and inexpensive' (Oudshoorn 1994: 73). The urine of pregnant mares was even less expensive than human urine and in the 1930s Dutch farmers could sell it to laboratories for prices equal to that of cows' milk, an economic trend, which as we have seen, has continued until the present day (Oudshoorn 1994: 65).

In the case of men's sex hormones, however, obtaining research materials proved more difficult. Ovaries were available because it was a common medical procedure to remove them, but as there was no similar operation for men, scientists had to wait for prison executions to obtain testes (Moscucci 1990: 134). In the case of urine, there were no institutions catering specifically to men's health that could collect it. Sick men's urine could not be used as the hormone levels were too low and animal urine also failed to provide the required amount of hormones. Police and military barracks and prisons were tried but difficulties remained, largely because such great amounts of urine were required to produce only milligrams of hormone.[3] Oudshoorn concludes, 'It was only when male sex hormones could be made synthetically [in 1936] and organic materials were no longer needed, that an increase took place in research on male sex hormones' (Oudshoorn 1994: 77).

Oudshoorn argues that this difference in accessibility of female and male gonads and urine had an important effect on the field of sex hormone research, helping to strengthen the role of gynaecologists in the field. Because gynaecologists had the easiest access to women's urine, the knowledge claims they attached to female sex hormones became stronger than the claims of the other groups, such as biochemists and physiologists. This meant 'claims concerning the role of female sex hormones in female disorders and female reproduction gained more momentum than claims concerning sexual differentiation and male reproductive functions'

---

[3] Oudshoorn reports the work of a German chemist who used 25,000 litres of urine from police barracks to produce 50 mg of crystalline hormone (Oudshoorn 1994: 76). The practical problems alone of collecting, transporting and working on these quantities of liquid were considerable.

(Oudshoorn 1994: 80). Pharmaceutical companies also became involved in matters pertaining to women's hormones at this time, as they played a critical role in supplying materials to laboratory scientists.

In January 1925 the Dutch company Organon put their first female sex hormone preparation on the market. This product had only been tested on five scientists at their laboratories. At this stage, Oudshoorn argues, 'Sex hormones could best be described as drugs looking for a market' (Oudshoorn 1994: 108). The hormones were tested as a treatment for menstrual disorders, with Organon supplying the medication free to gynaecological clinics in exchange for the women's urine needed to make the product. In less than two years, the proposed applications of female sex hormones had increased far beyond menstrual disorders. In a 1927 advertisement Organon recommended hormone therapy for 'all anomalies of ovarian function, causing disorders in menstruation and other sexual functions in women, in particular retardation in growth of the genital organs leading to sterility and in cases of menopausal complaints' (cited in Oudshoorn 1994: 93). Hormone-therapy usage was also extended to the psychiatric clinic, where female sex hormones were tested as treatments for depression and psychoses attributed to menstrual disorders. The net for hormone therapy was spread even wider in 1929 when ailments such as epilepsy, hair loss, eye disorders, diabetes, haemophilia and chilblained feet were included as indications for such treatment.

Inconclusive test results and the sheer range and vagueness of these indications led Organon, in conjunction with gynaecological clinics, to organise large-scale trials of the effects of female sex hormones on menopausal symptoms. During the 1930s, menopause was increasingly studied and came to be seen as a deficiency of sex hormones (Bell 1987). This construction was beneficial to pharmaceutical companies as they could promote their treatment as a remedy for such deficiency. In 1938, then, Organon chose menopause as the major medical indication for female sex hormones, although menstrual disorders were also still seen as important (Oudshoorn 1994: 94–6).

In contrast to this picture of pharmaceutical companies tapping into existing structures (gynaecology clinics) to promote hormone therapy for women, there were no clinics dealing with men's problems and no obvious places to set up clinical trials.[4] Also the memory of Brown-Séquard's claims about renewed sexual vigour, and the consequent 'quackery'

---

[4] The speciality of andrology was established in the USA in the 1970s (Clarke 1998: 40; see also Moscucci 1990).

surrounding monkey gland and other preparations, made scientists and pharmaceutical companies reluctant to trial the effects of male sex hormones on aging men (Hirschbein 2000). Male sex-hormone therapy was used to treat prostate hypertrophy and depression and melancholy, but did not develop into a widely applicable treatment. Oudshoorn claims this lack of an institutional base and network spelt the failure of male HRT.[5]

One area in which male hormonal medications were used was in 'treating' homosexuals, which may also have had a negative impact on the development of HRT for aging men. Male hormones were used as a 'treatment' of male homosexuals in the 1930s and 1940s, especially in the United States. The recipients of these 'treatments' were usually men who had been arrested for sexual or other offences (Terry 1999: 268–96). The procedures were singularly ineffectual and were in the main superseded by psychoanalytic and behaviourist approaches, although their use continued well into the second half of the twentieth century (Terry 1999: 162–3).

In Chapter 1, I discussed Oudshoorn's social-network analysis and suggested that other less immediately relevant networks intersect or cross over the technoscientific networks described in her history of endocrinology. Using Serres' notion of crumpled time, I argued that older understandings and concepts are commonly folded into technoscience, largely through the embodiment of scientists and other actors, but also through non-human actors such as medical and scientific technologies. Building on this argument, the following section analyses the historically significant conceptions of racial and sexual differences that were folded into HRT technologies as they developed over the twentieth century.

Scientific theories of sexual and racial differences

In *The Second Sex*, de Beauvoir describes menopausal women as falling outside the binary distinction of sex. 'It is sometimes said', she writes, 'that women of a certain age constitute "a third sex"; and, in truth, while they are not males, they are no longer females' (de Beauvoir 1988: 63). This quote reveals the problem posed by the menopause for twentieth-century understandings of sexual difference: the loss of sexual differences associated with aging creates significant confusion for understandings of sex based on reproductivity. If women are no longer reproductive after menopause, can

---

[5] Oudshoorn's more recent book, *The Male Pill: A biography of a technology in the making* (2003) tells a fascinating related story about multiple failed attempts to create and distribute a male contraceptive pill.

they still be understood as women? Similarly for men: if reproductive penetrative sex is no longer possible for older males, are they still men?

Early twentieth-century endocrinologists were somewhat perplexed when faced with a developing understanding of sex hormones that confounded the two-sex model of differences between men and women. Social changes brought about by feminist and homosexual movements, as well as the theories and therapeutic practices of sexology and psychoanalysis, were also simultaneously challenging social, psychological and physiological understandings of masculinity and femininity and the biologically sexed body. The two-sex model, however, was not overturned by endocrinological discoveries. Rather, biomedical and technoscientific discourses worked to accommodate new data, developing a model of a sexual continuum in which healthy, ideal men and women occupy 'opposite' ends of a spectrum whilst pathological 'others' take up the places in-between. Thus, for example, rather than constituting a 'third sex' *outside* a binary distinction, menopausal women are understood as simply *closer* to men than healthy, reproductive women.[6] This closeness is described in terms of aging women's reduced femininity, but also, in places, in terms of their increased physical – rather than sexual – virility (increased facial hair and male pattern baldness, for example). Hierarchies also pervade this continuum: as many feminist theorists have argued, the male or masculine end of the continuum within a two-sex model is valued more highly and indeed, is figured as a healthy norm against which other bodies are measured and found to be lacking (see, for example, LeDoeuff 1989).

Numerous historians have suggested that modern understandings of the sexes as opposite and/or complementary were intertwined with discourses on racial differences.[7] Nancy Leys Stepan (1993) argues, for example, that the nineteenth-century focus on binary sexual difference was partially enabled by an analogy made between sexual difference and racial difference, whereby supposed deficiencies were found in both European women and non-European people of both sexes. The analogy between sex and race, Stepan demonstrates, was supported by evolutionary discourse in which European women's inferior position in relation to European men was explained by their retention of features of 'primitive races' (Stepan 1993: 360; see also Stepan and Gilman 1993). Philosopher Sally Markowitz

---

[6] The model of a hormonal life-course from Reinisch *et al.* (1991) discussed in Chapter 3 indicates this conception of aging as involving a loss of hormonal difference between the sexes.

[7] See, for example, Gilman 1985, 1991, 1993; Russett 1989; Stepan 1993; Stepan and Gilman 1993; Takaki 1993.

(2001) extends this argument, suggesting that the two-sex model was always dependent on notions of racial hierarchy. She analyses the writings of turn-of-the-century British sexologist Havelock Ellis to demonstrate this dependency. Whilst Havelock Ellis is generally regarded as one of the more radical British sexologists of his time, Markowitz shows that his theories of sexual difference relied on and reinforced racial hierarchies.[8] Ellis' argument regarding sexual and racial differences focused on feminine beauty and, in particular, on the beauty of the 'generous pelvis' (Markowitz 2001: 393). The pelvis – as foreshadowed by the earlier anatomists analysed by Londa Schiebinger (1989) – represented women's ability to give birth. For Ellis, the fact that white women's pelvises were wider than those of non-white women demonstrated they had developed to allow for the birth of the larger-brained, and hence superior, white child (Markowitz 2001: 393).

In focussing on pelvises, Ellis centres questions of racial and sexual difference on issues of sexuality and reproduction. Markowitz shows that Ellis' theories of sexuality distinguish between the periodic sex drives of 'savages' and the more reproduction-focused 'psychic' sexuality expressed by white Europeans. Female domesticity, maternal feeling and beauty – the key elements of Ellis' two-sex model – are all linked to a particular version of white European bourgeois culture. This focus on white women's reproductive capacities, Markowitz argues, allowed colonialists to reduce anxieties around miscegenation rising from their relations with non-western women and to argue the rightfulness of white supremacy (Markowitz 2001: 400–1). Markowitz thus concludes that 'the ideology of sex/gender difference itself turns out to rest ... on a scale of racially coded degrees of sex/gender difference culminating in the manly European man and the feminine European woman' (Markowitz 2001: 391).

Sex hormones and women's 'natural' pathologies

These ideas about sexual and racial differences were mobilised within scientific work on hormones and HRT.[9] Tests developed in the 1930s to establish levels of hormones in the blood, for example, allowed

---

[8] In addition, Jeffrey Weeks (1981: 149–53) argues that Ellis' work was conservative in relation to its focus on reproductive heterosexuality and its ultimate dependence on arguing the existence of a basic biological impulse towards reproduction.

[9] Other arguments made about the hormonal bases of racial and sexual differences referred to the adrenal glands and thyroid function. In 1935, for example, Jennie Gregory's *ABC of the*

endocrinologists to describe male and female bodies as fundamentally different in terms of cyclicity and stability. Through these synchronic assessments of hormone levels, 'The female body became characterised by its cyclic hormonal regulation and the male body by its stable hormonal regulation' (Oudshoorn 1994: 146). This new view of sexual difference was attached to older understandings of women as essentially reproductive. The development of hormonal tests (for pregnancy, for example) and treatments (hormone-replacement therapies, for example) allowed the medical profession to intervene in reproduction cycles, 'thus', Oudshoorn argues, 'bringing the "natural" features of reproduction and aging into the domain of medical intervention' (Oudshoorn 1994: 147–8). Chemical cyclicity, in other words, came to figure as physiological evidence of women's difference, a figuration that opened up a spectrum of hormonal treatment options to regulate these cycles.

Figuring cyclicity as a natural difference between men and women caused conceptual problems regarding the cessation of menstruation at menopause. In line with their adherence to synchronic analyses of life, scientists and clinicians queried why this natural difference should end. Feminist science-studies theorist Bernice Hausman argues that this question necessitated an understanding of menopause 'as a malfunction, rather than a change in function or the cessation of an unnecessary function' (Hausman 1995: 33). By the 1950s, then, menopause came to be seen as an unnecessary and pathological disruption to natural sexual difference.[10]

Within this model of menopause as pathology, HRT could be presented as facilitating the maintenance of a thereby naturalised femininity. This understanding of HRT as providing hormones to maintain 'natural' femininity was further developed in the 1960s when HRT became a popular pharmaceutical product, fiercely promoted by gynaecologist Robert A. Wilson (McCrea 1983; Bell 1987). Wilson's *Feminine Forever* suggested that women should take oestrogen from their mid-thirties until death in

Endocrines, described the 'facial contours' of the 'Mongoloid and negro' as due to 'hypofunction' of the thyroid (Gregory 1935: 94). In the same year, Ivo Geiko Cobb published *The Glands of Destiny (A Study of the Personality)*, which argued that different racial 'types' were dominated by different hormones (Cobb 1935: 146). In 1921, Louis Berman had also argued that European women of the 'adrenal type' were 'always masculinoid'. If adrenal activity was not balanced by other hormones, he warned, viewers would 'behold the maiden aunts, the prudes and the cranks who never satisfactorily adapt themselves in society' (Berman, cited in Donovan 1988: 8). The adrenal gland, then, was associated with white masculinity: a noble characteristic that was denied to black and Asian men and seen as undesirable in women.

[10] See, Hausman 1995: 32–4; Leysen 1996: 176–7; Martin 1997: 242; Sybylla 1997: 211.

order to avoid menopause, which he described as intolerable castration: 'Because the chemical balance of the entire organism is disrupted', Wilson (1966: 37) wrote, 'menopausal castration amounts to a mutilation of the whole body'. As is clear in his title, Wilson unashamedly linked oestrogen with femininity: like de Beauvoir, he states that menopausal women 'are no longer women' (Wilson 1966: 39). The femininity restored by HRT is a culturally specific one: in *Feminine Forever*, Wilson provides as much (strong) opinion on proper sexual behaviour, dress and marriage, as on biological or medical factors.

Wilson's work was taken up by many other doctors, especially in the United States and was excerpted widely in popular magazines throughout the 1960s and 1970s. The idea that menopause constituted the loss of sexual difference was explicit in these popular works. In the best-selling 1969 book, *Everything You Always Wanted to Know about Sex*, for example, psychiatrist David Reuben describes the menopausal woman as neither 'a functional woman' nor a man:

> As the oestrogen is shut off, a woman comes as close as she can to being a man. Increased facial hair, deepened voice, obesity, and decline of breasts and female genitalia all contribute to a masculine appearance. Coarsened features, enlargement of the clitoris, and a gradual baldness complete the tragic picture. Not really a man but no longer a functional woman, these individuals live in a world of intersex.
>
> *(Reuben 1971: 315)*

'Having outlived their ovaries', Reuben (1971: 316) concludes, 'they have outlived their usefulness as human beings.'

This elision between loss of sexual difference and loss of humanity resonates with Shippen's desire to 'put a stake through the ugly little heart' of the male menopause. Like Shippen's more recent menopausal man, Reuben's menopausal woman is an outcast of society, a 'useless' being. The mobilisation of such strong rhetoric to persuade aging people to take medication to prevent hormonal decline is insidious and, unsurprisingly perhaps, powerful.

As many feminists have argued, these intense campaigns marketing HRT to women were highly successful. By the mid-1970s, enormous amounts of hormone-replacement therapy were being prescribed in the United States and although numbers declined in the later 1970s due to links made between hormonal treatment and cancer, high levels of prescriptions continued to the turn of the century. Having dropped to approximately 15 million prescriptions per year in 1979–80, HRT prescriptions in the United States were up to nearly 32 million per year in 1989 (Worcester and Whatley 1992: 4) and to 68 million by 2000 (Fletcher and Colditz 2002). In Britain, rates of HRT usage have always been lower than in the United States, nevertheless 6 million prescriptions were issued in England alone in 2001 (Ellerington, Whitcroft and Whitehead 1992; Hill 2002). In Australia rates of usage of 58 per cent amongst target groups were reached in the mid-1990s (MacLennan, Taylor and Wilson 1995), whilst in Germany, 25 per cent of women aged 40–69 were taking HRT in 1991 (Oddens *et al.* 1992). In Scandinavia, turn-of-the-century usage rates ranged from 9 per cent in Oslo to 32 per cent in Helsinki (European HRT–Network Foundation 2001).

Importantly, promotion of HRT in pharmaceutical advertising and the popular media continues to represent HRT as providing or boosting 'femininity' (Coney 1991; Roberts 2002a). In recent features in the tabloid press in Britain, for example, photographed ultra-feminine celebrities enthusiastically affirm the benefits of HRT (Hope 2002: 19; Marsh 2002: 30; Finnegan 2002: 15). Describing the menopause in her regular social commentary column, well-known *Daily Express* commentator and TV personality Judy Finnegan writes, 'We all feel that this great watershed deprives us of something central to our femaleness. With the end of our fertile days, we worry we'll kiss goodbye to sexual desire, allure and femininity' (Finnegan 2002: 15).[11] The solution to this loss is simple for Finnegan. 'HRT has transformed women's lives', she asserts, advising her readers that 'If you think you need it, make sure you get it' (Finnegan 2002: 15).[12]

The menopause as unnatural difference

Many medical, pharmaceutical and popular discourses represent menopause as a pathology that signals the end of femininity and thus requires medication. In so doing, HRT discourses invoke a two-sex model of sexual

---

[11] Judy Finnegan and Richard Maddley form 'Britain's best-loved husband and wife team' (Maddley and Finnegan 2002: 14), hosting a television chat show 'Richard and Judy' and writing a weekly editorial on current events in the *Daily Express*.

[12] As discussed in Chapter 5, comments like these took on a new biopolitical edge after the premature cessation of the world's largest clinical trial of HRT in May 2002. Rather than proving the positive qualities of HRT, this trial indicated that HRT increases risk of heart disease and other serious health conditions. This news produced both a serious global decline in HRT prescriptions and a consequent flurry of media articles, like that cited here, in which famous women asserted their continued belief in the powers of this medication. It also led to the closure of hundreds of urine-producing stables in North America – a fact that has further inflamed the animal rights debates surrounding Premarin[TM] and led to attempts to rehome the 20,000 now 'redundant' mares and their foals (Morrison 2004).

difference in which femininity is inextricably linked to reproductivity. In explaining the pathological menopause, however, some contemporary medical literature goes even further, arguing that menopause is essentially *unnatural*. It is in this figuration of the menopause that ideas of racial difference enter HRT discourses most powerfully.

A letter published in the *British Medical Journal* provides an example of this view. In the following quotation, gynaecologist Kim Hinshaw (1996) uses the notion of the unnaturalness of menopause (its non-physiological nature) to counter concerns about the promotion of HRT to women, arguing that western women today live in a pathological state of 'socially-induced longevity'. Some authors, he writes,

> consider the menopause to be physiological and hormone replacement therapy to be a drug that should not be offered to a general population. This view requires the belief that an event that potentially affects all women must be part of the normal aging process. This fact alone is not irrefutable evidence that the menopause is a physiological process. This century, average female life expectancy has risen from 45 to 83 years. This is almost entirely related to considerable improvements in social conditions and means that a woman may now spend almost one third of her life in the postmenopausal state ... Perhaps we can regard the menopause as the onset of a pathological state to which women are exposed only because of socially induced longevity.
>
> *(Hinshaw 1996: 686)*

The notion of the unnatural or non-physiological menopause is supported by a 'fact' deemed inexplicable if menopause were understood as physiological: non-western women do not suffer from menopause to anything like the extent western women do (see, for example, Boulet *et al.* 1994). This fact leads medical scientists to search for explanations of menopause that lie outside the realms of endocrinology, a search often leading to the claim made above by Hinshaw, that menopause as demonstrated by western women is socially or environmentally, rather than biologically, caused. As will be demonstrated below, such explanations in turn rely on assertions that non-western women lead more natural lives and therefore do not require HRT.

In late twentieth-century discussions of HRT and menopause, understandings of the necessity for HRT for most western women is entwined both with racist views of the lives of non-western and poor women and with a privileging of a binary and narrow understanding of sexual differences. The contemporary development of HRT for men also relies on narrow views of sexual, class and racial differences. In this view, femininity is seen to be about reproduction, receptive sex and physical beauty and masculinity about penetrative sex and physical strength. In both cases, HRT is figured as providing support for these characteristics that, although natural (seen to be occurring 'naturally' in non-western populations), are failing in the west due to environmental conditions.

A special issue of the *British Medical Bulletin* on HRT published in 1992 provides an example of these arguments. Although most of the articles focus only on western women and on specific information about HRT, the final article by osteoporosis researcher J. Reeve, entitled 'Future Prospects for Hormone Replacement Therapy', contrasts western and non-western women's experiences of menopause. Reeve begins by listing the 'principal adverse consequences' of the menopause, stating that these 'relate to its effects on the cardiovascular system and the skeleton' (Reeve 1992: 459). In the next sentences, however, he notes that these effects appear to be limited largely to affluent western populations: '[W]ith regard to the cardiovascular system and the skeleton', he writes,

> evidence that menopause leads to significant adverse health consequences
> comes largely from studies on affluent, westernized populations. Whereas
> postmenopausal bone loss appears to occur at similar rates in African as in
> European populations, there is evidence that age-adjusted rates of serious
> insufficiency fractures are at least an order of magnitude lower in some African
> populations. Likewise, cardiovascular disease ... occurs at much lower rates
> in many third world than in typical western postmenopausal populations.
> Oriental populations also have lower rates.
>
> *(Reeve 1992: 459)*

In trying to explain these differences, Reeve points not to biological differences between western and non-western women, but to environmental factors:

> [T]rends in both osteoporotic fractures and myocardial disease evident over
> the last three decades in most western countries point to important environ-
> mental influences over these disorders.
>
> *(Reeve 1992: 459)*

Indeed, Reeve argues that the worsening rates of osteoporotic fractures and heart disease in western women 'have little to do with the hormonal status of the women affected' (Reeve 1992: 459). Accordingly, biological measures of risk of osteoporosis or heart disease, he adds, are not transferable from western to non-western populations:

> Nor can simple clinical measurements, such as cholesterol levels or bone
> density indices, be used as measures of risk that can, for example, be transferred
> from an affluent western population to a third world population.
>
> *(Reeve 1992: 459)*

According to Reeve, then, the experience of menopause as causing fractures and/or heart disease is confined to western women. Surprisingly, this does not lead to suggestions for environmental or social change but to the recommendation of HRT for western women only. 'Accordingly', Reeve writes, 'HRT is more likely to promote women's health in affluent westernized cultures than in third world subsistence cultures' (Reeve 1992: 459). The reference to non-western women's lower rates of osteoporosis and heart disease, in other words, does not ultimately disrupt the medical, hormonal model. Instead, reference to non-western women functions to support the recommendation to prescribe HRT to affluent western women and to deem its use by women in 'third world subsistence cultures' unnecessary.[13]

In Reeve's argument, to summarise, pathological menopause is understood as non-biological. This claim is linked to the idea that women in developing countries do not experience pathological menopause and do not, therefore, require HRT. Thus, the menopause, which is normally understood to be biological, is held to be environmental and at the same time, non-western women's lives are figured as 'natural'.

A second example comes from gynaecologist and medical anthropologist Joel Wilbush, who in a series of articles spanning almost two decades, argues that menopausal difficulties are environmentally rather than biologically produced.[14] Wilbush's statements about the menopause (or 'climacteric') rely on a similar argument to that offered by Reeves. 'Western women's climacteric ills', he writes, 'are primarily due to the stresses to which society and the culture had, in the past, subjected them and, in many ways still continue to do so' (Wilbush 1994: 342). Attempting to provide a contrast to this pathogenic western way of life, Wilbush asks 'How and in what way does a modern civilized woman then differ from a "natural" woman?' (Wilbush 1994: 344). His answer refers to four groups of 'natural' women:

As far as it is possible to conjecture female *Homo erectus*, or early sapiens, even women in preindustrial societies and many today, share one basic feature: they were and are, most of their lives, either pregnant or breast feeding. Modern Western women are not and do not, instead they menstruate.

(Wilbush 1994: 344)

[13] No recommendation is made regarding those 'oriental populations' who have lower rates of heart disease but presumably do not fit within the category of 'third world subsistence cultures'.

[14] See Wilbush 1981a, 1981b, 1985, 1988a, 1988b, 1993, 1994. In 2002, the Hebrew University inaugurated the Wilbush Chair of Medical Anthropology to facilitate research on evolution and human aging.

Developing this contrast, Wilbush goes on to cite other reasons why western women today are unnatural. In particular, the use of contraception, 'especially when not effected through hormonal oral contraception ... results in incessant ovulation', which is 'almost always harmful' (Wilbush 1994: 344). It is this incessant ovulation (which he names 'a product of Western social conditions') that is held to cause menopausal symptoms and many other diseases, such as cervical and uterine cancer.

This set of claims leads Wilbush to argue that western women should take HRT to help them through their unnatural situation. After his list of diseases to which western women are subject, he adds:

> These lists of woes are not intended to frighten, nor persuade women to have long strings of children; that would be a global catastrophe. For surely women consider the gains they have made well worth the price. The benefits of civilization, so greatly helped by hormonal medication, far outweigh the 'state of nature', even if it means a small measure of medical intervention. Is the cost of medical advice really so high?
>
> *(Wilbush 1994: 344)*

Wilbush thus proposes that all western women take HRT in an attempt to 'eliminate' their unnatural menopause. 'Since a "menopausal crisis", or even recognition of the cessation of the menses as stressful, is ... not a natural process, there seems little to gain by protesting its artificial elimination' (Wilbush 1994: 344).

In contrast to his representation of such unnecessary protests, Wilbush suggests that western women are rightly concerned with the effects of the 'unnatural' menopause on their appearance. Indeed, he suggests that 'the waning of female attractiveness ... [is] the only *real* loss most Western women have repeatedly and so keenly felt' and argues that this desire to remain physically attractive constitutes women's genetic difference from men (Wilbush 1994: 345). When linked with his view of the menopause as unnatural, this claim of women's concerns with beauty being genetic constitutes a paradox (technically, a chiasmas).[15] What might be thought to be natural (and what many feminists have argued is natural) – the menopause – is positioned as unnatural. At the same time, what is generally thought to be social – the fact that women are expected to be concerned with their appearance and sexual attractiveness – is positioned as genetic.[16]

[15] I analyse the chiastic structure of this argument in Roberts 2003a.
[16] This emphasis on women's appearance as a sign of sexual difference has a long history. Ellis refers to it in detail, as do other nineteenth-century writers. Discussion of women's appearance was common in the medical literature about menopause at least up until the

Wilbush's logic is used to support the recommendation of HRT to western women: through 'eliminating' the unnatural menopause, taking HRT prevents the loss of women's natural difference (beauty). Feminist arguments against HRT are dismissed within Wilbush's argument as an illogical attempt to defend an unnatural state and puritanically to refuse women's desire to preserve a natural one. Wilbush's work demonstrates the ways in which 'nature', signifying a desired form of health, can become attached to a pharmaceutical product. 'Nature', in his logic, has shifting value and conveys enormous historical freight in terms of its connections to both sexual and racial differences.

Racial differences and the politics of reproduction

As in Havelock Ellis' writings, Wilbush's view of sexual difference is dependent upon a particular understanding of racial differences. His vision of the unnatural western women needing HRT depends on a fantasy of the natural, non-western woman living a life of continuous reproduction. But how does this connection get played out in contemporary biomedical discourses around the menopause and HRT?

Today, biomedical discourses constituting the field of women's health are increasingly attempting to take account of some differences amongst women. In contraceptive technology discourses, for example, Oudshoorn suggests that differences amongst white women in the west are beginning to be acknowledged. These women are now more frequently offered a range of contraceptive technologies, in what is called the 'cafeteria' approach (Oudshoorn 1996a, 1996b; see also Clarke 1998: 204). Racial differences, however, Oudshoorn argues, frequently remain negated or reduced. 'Although the cafeteria discourse has disrupted the former scientific representations of the gendered subject-object relations', she writes, 'it has reinforced the othering of people of colour' (Oudshoorn 1996b: 167). This is evidenced by the fact that hormonal contraceptives are tested in non-western countries, assuming that non-western women can be used as reliable stand-ins for western women. As well, women in non-western countries (and some women of colour in western countries) are not offered the same level of contraceptive choice as white women. Some are forced to use particular contraceptive technologies, while others are the targets of directed governmental campaigns 'offering' one technology much more strongly than

early 1980s. These texts emphasised the importance of women maintaining their physical appearance after menopause as central to their health (Kaufert 1982).

others.[17] These differences are linked to western fears of population growth and its effect on environmental degradation and to desires to facilitate the control of the birth rates of particular groups of people.[18]

As shown above, some contemporary medical discourses suggest that non-western women do not need HRT because they live natural lives. Debates and practices around contraception, however, demonstrate that these natural lives have long been figured as problematic because they produce 'too many' children. Many non-western and poor women are subjected to the most invasive contraceptive technologies in order to curb their reproductivity. Wilbush's and Reeves' visions of the natural non-western woman, then, do not correlate with many contemporary women's experiences.[19] Contrasting natural non-western women and unnatural western women and assuming that non-western women would not benefit from HRT are both illogical lines of argument.

Analysing HRT discourses highlights how notions of racial and class differences are entangled with contemporary versions of the two-sex model. The construction of menopause as unnatural interlinks with the figuration of a particular version of binary sexual difference as natural. This figuration centres on women's reproductivity and is supported by racist and classist fantasies of non-western and economically deprived women's reproductive lives.

The version of binary sexual difference in operation in contemporary HRT discourses in which menopause is figured as a pathology stems from the two-sex model. As Markowitz demonstrates in her reading of Ellis, the two-sex model has always been intertwined with hierarchical understandings of racial differences. Markowitz argues that this systematic connection between versions of sexual difference and hierarchical racial ideologies remains overlooked in much contemporary feminist work on sex and gender. My analysis begins to address this oversight in relation to discourses around femininity and the menopause, but what about HRT discourses aimed at men?

---

[17] See, for example, Hardon 1992; Doyal 1995; Oudshoorn 1996b and the essays in Russell, Sobo and Thompson 2000.

[18] See, for example, LaCheen 1986; Bunkle 1997; Doyal 1995; Russell and Thompson 2000.

[19] The vision of the 'natural' constantly childbearing woman also fails to correlate with what is known about women in indigenous societies *before* they were subjected to western culture and contraceptive technologies. In precolonisation Aboriginal cultures in Australia, for example, childbearing was successfully controlled by various means. Birth rates amongst Aboriginal women increased greatly *after* colonisation (Cowlishaw 1982).

HRT for men: a new model of sexual difference?

In his 1991 editorial, geriatrician John Morely opines that

> Should testosterone eventually prove useful to improve muscle strength in the elderly, we in medicine may need to ponder why it will have taken more than 100 years since Brown-Séquard's report, which showed a 6- to 7-kg increase in forearm strength, for this therapy to become readily available to our patients.
>
> *(Morely 1991: 897)*

This is an unusually positive reference to late nineteenth-century endocrinological history. Citing Brown-Séquard's hard data, Morely bypasses the more uncomfortable associations of this work (elaborated in the so-called monkey gland affair) and folds this early research into contemporary technoscience. This resuscitation of 100-year-old data is part of a concerted effort to promote an 'old' medication that provokes new questions about the semiotic materialities of sexed bodies today: does the move towards providing hormonal supplementation of masculine embodiment (specifically muscular strength, leanness and bone mass) and penetrative sex drive mean a moving away from the two-sex model of sexual difference? And does it mean, finally, an acknowledgement of *both* sexes as differentiated and embodied, rather than the positioning of only women as (pathologically) different? Or is it rather, recognition that 'natural' sexual differences require chemical supplementation in aging women *and* men?

The development of HRT for men needs to be considered not only within the broader context of contemporary bio-sociality, but also in relation to what some social theorists have called a 'crisis' of masculinity, a series of significant changes in experiences and representations of masculinity or maleness.[20] The (re)development of hormone replacement for men is part of these broad trends. The change is also strongly affected by the often-announced fact that western populations in general are aging: that there will be in the next century significantly more older people than ever before. The combination of these three fields (bio-sociality, the 'crisis' in masculinity and the expansion of aging) has produced an appealing new market for pharmaceutical and biomedical products. Cosmetic surgery and anti-impotence medication are two areas with which male HRT is linked.

Cultural theorist Margaret Morganroth Gullette (1994) argues that in contemporary American culture aging men's bodies are positioned as

---

[20] See, for example, Berger, Wallis and Watson 1995; Connell 2000; Whitehead and Barrett 2001; Nye 2005.

problematic and in need of supplementation. In an analysis of cartoons, popular media and statistics about men using hair dyes, cosmetics and other articles designed to help fight the appearance of aging, Gullette shows that the gap between men and women in relation to a problematisation of aging is closing (see also Gullette 2004). The growing numbers of men using cosmetic surgery to change signs of aging is also testament to this.[21] Other theorists make similar points, but argue that significant differences remain between the experiences of men and women. In relation to cosmetic surgery, for example, Anne Balsamo demonstrates how advertisements for such surgery aimed at men emphasise the need for men to look younger in order to maintain and improve their positions at work. This is a rather different emphasis to those aimed at women, which focus on the inherent imperfections of women's bodies (Balsamo 1996: 67–71). The increasing number of men using cosmetic surgery does not indicate equivalence, Balsamo argues, between cultural imaginations of men's and women's aging bodies:

> The codes that structure cosmetic surgery advertising are gendered in stereotypical ways: being male requires a concern with virility and productivity, whereas being a real woman requires buying beauty products and services ... The naturalized identity of the female body as pathological and diseased is culturally reproduced in media discussions and representations of cosmetic surgery services.
>
> *(Balsamo 1996: 70–1)*

Kathleen Woodward (1991, 1994) makes a similar point in her work on aging. Although she is concerned not to subordinate the youth/age distinction to sexual difference, she maintains that there are important differences in experiences and representations of aging for men and women. She argues that as the number of older people increases in America, in many ways they become less visible. Encouraged to live together in retirement villages somewhat removed from other generations, older people are also advised to masquerade youth through cosmetic surgery, diets and exercise programmes. These masquerade practices, however, are connected more strongly to women – a fact that reflects a long association of women with masquerade and the notion that women are or need to be more concerned with their appearance. As well, Woodward writes, 'Women are *aged by society* earlier than are men' (Woodward 1994: 61). This is evident in discussions of postmenopausal women's use of reproductive technologies. Such discussions evidence a strong cultural discomfort with older women

---

[21] See Gullette 1994: 228–9: Davis 1995; Balsamo 1996: 67–71; Fraser 2003: 74–5.

having babies, a discomfort that is not equalled when older men have children with younger women.

The anti-impotence medication Viagra provides another example of the ways in which biomedical products are used to address physical problems of aging. Sold to men as a quick and painless solution to erectile dysfunction, this medication reproduces heteronormative and normatively youthful sexual 'scripts'.[22] Viagra supports a particular form of sexual practice – penetration of the vagina by the penis – figured as essential to healthy life. Punning on Wilson's 'feminine forever', Barbara Marshall and Stephen Katz (2002) argue that Viagra discourses promise aging men they will remain 'forever functional'. Laura Mamo and Jennifer Fishman (2001: 26–7) also find that Viagra advertisements produce a racialised Viagra user, always representing racially 'homogenous' couples.

HRT for men combines elements of discourses on cosmetic surgery and Viagra by promising to sustain a particular vision and experience of the male body as muscular *and* sexually active in particular ways (i.e., having penetrative sex at what is deemed by doctors to be an acceptable frequency). Biomedical articles about HRT promise that 'Evidence shows that most men treated with testosterone will feel better about themselves and their lives' (Bain 2001: 91). In these discourses, sex hormones are linked to youth (and therefore life itself) via sexuality. Men are described as needing testosterone replacement because 'frequency of intercourse decreases with age' (Morely 1991: 86) as impotence increases. This is seen to be a disaster by geriatricians such as Morely because, as he quotes, 'Aging is regarded as a demon that heralds approaching death, whereas sex is equated with life ... sexuality is especially significant for an older person's morale [because] it is an affirmation of life and a denial of death' (Dean, quoted in Morely 1991: 84). Such affirmation is figured as important for men, who are expected to want penetrative sex even into their second century (see Kaiser 1991: 68).[23] As geriatrician Fran Kaiser writes, despite the fact that 55 per cent of men are impotent by the age of 75 (i.e., they cannot 'obtain an erection adequate for intercourse in 75 per cent or more of attempts' or they never make attempts), this impotence 'should not be considered part of the normal aging process' (Kaiser 1991: 63). If impotence were accepted as part of the 'normal aging process', definitions

---

[22] See, for example, Mamo and Fishman 2001; Marshall 2002; Marshall and Katz 2002; Katz and Marshall 2003; Potts *et al.* 2003; Potts 2004.

[23] Kaiser (1991: 68) writes, 'Sexual problems in older ages (80- to 102-year-olds) include fear of poor performance and impotence, and lack of opportunity for sexual encounters.'

of male subjectivity and embodiment would have to be rethought. Such rethinking would require a move away from a synchronic analysis of the actions of sex hormones to a diachronic one – one that could take positive account of physical change over a man's lifetime, rather than relying on a static model of sexual identity that positions all change as pathological decline. Rather than introducing such a model into studies of aging, contemporary gerontology prefers to promote HRT, Viagra and penile implants as supplements for a narrow version of male sexuality. Such supplementation, as mentioned earlier, is also potentially highly profitable; aging men, like menopausal women, represent a massive and ever-increasing market that, if it becomes anxious enough, promises dreamy profits to pharmaceutical companies (see Katz and Marshall 2003).

The pathological loss of masculinity constituting contemporary forms of male aging has only very recently been scientifically linked with decreases in testosterone.[24] The necessity for testosterone replacement, then, remains unstable in the medical literature, although, as cited earlier, some clinicians are promoting its 'aggressive' application. The connection between declining levels of testosterone and the physical and mental changes of aging will require significant medical and popular promotion before they are widely accepted. In recent North American and Euopean studies, aging men demonstrated a poor knowledge of the andropause and its hormonal correlates (Solstad and Garde 1992; Tan and Philip 1999). In an American study of 302 'older males', many experienced symptoms of andropause (impotence, weakness and memory loss), but most did not understand this as an endocrinopathy (Tan and Philip 1999). The majority (70 per cent) expressed an interest in acquiring further knowledge regarding andropause, however. The promise that 'most men treated with testosterone will feel better about themselves and their lives' (Bain 2001: 91) is one that many men may well take seriously.

Pharmaceutical advertising for male HRT messages a narrow version of masculine embodiment: the man taking Androderm^{TM}, for example, is symbolised in advertisements published in medical journals as a naked and muscular golden god standing in a circle, legs spread, arms firing a large arrow into the air in imitation of the traditional male symbol (Watson Pharma Inc. 1996). The andropausal man is also figured in medical and popular discourses as an individual – his experiences of pathological aging are not inevitable or natural (like those of the menopausal woman), but

---

[24] See Kaufman and Vermeulen 1997; Morales *et al.* 1997; Vermeulen 2000; Morely 2000, 2001; Bain 2001.

specific to each particular case. 'Contrary to menopause in women', one medical article suggests, 'andropause is not an obligatory event in men, and when it does occur, its pathogenesis and hormonal aspects are very variable' (Mastrogiacomo *et al.* 1982: 293). Another argues that '"Andropause" or "male climacteric" refer to the term "menopause" in women. The parallelism between both entities is however only partial, since the decrease of gonadal function in the male is very different from one individual to another' (Legros 2000: 449). This emphasis on the individuality of andro-pausal men and on the gradual rather than sudden decline of sex hormones in aging men (in contrast to the sudden decline of oestrogens in women) promotes a masculinist (literally phallocentric) view of hormones' sex messaging. Unlike aging women, who are all pathological, andropausal men have individual problems that may be solved by HRT. Through testosterone replacement, men can be restored to their god-like embodi-ment of the healthy norm (what the Androderm™ advertisement calls 'the physiological ideal').

Reproduction is also central to the differential figurations of aging men and women and the sex messaging involved in HRT. It is commonly emphasised in the andropause literature that declining testosterone levels in men do not produce infertility as a norm of aging. As Vermeulen writes:

> In contrast to women, fertility in men persists until a very old age. However, testicular function of both the exo- and endocrine compartments decreases in old age, causing a series of clinical symptoms which are analogous to, although less pronounced than, the menopausal syndrome. These symptoms can be considered to represent the male climacterium or andropause. However, whereas at menopause ovarian hormonal secretion ceases almost completely, the decrease in the levels of biologically active androgens (free testosterone) is only moderate and many elderly men have free androgen levels that would be considered normal for young men.
>
> *(Vermeulen 1993: 531)*

The connections between women's 'natural' function of reproduction – the loss of which at menopause renders a woman 'no longer female' (de Beauvoir 1988: 63) – and oestrogen production is not mirrored in men. Most men are understood to maintain their 'natural' fertility, even though declines in libido and penetrative ability may not allow them to exercise it.[25] Thus testosterone replacement restores a (reproductive, hetero-) sexual norm in men in a way that is impossible in women.

---

[25] Studies increasingly report that men's fertility also declines with age (see, for example, Zavos *et al.* 2006). Other research, discussed in Chapter 6, describes declines in sperm quantity and quality in younger men in North America and Europe.

It is in relation to reproduction that racial arguments about HRT for men may develop, as the connections between reproductivity, race and testosterone have already been made. In a paper published in *Psychological Reports*, for example, Richard Lynn argues that 'Negroid' men have higher levels of testosterone than 'Caucasian' men, who in turn have higher levels than 'Mongoloid' men (Lynn 1990). These higher levels of testosterone are seen to cause increased sexual drive and sexual activity, which produce more children. This is analysed by Lynn as evidence of the impact of physiology on what are called 'reproduction strategies'. Negroid men are argued to be more reliant on an 'r strategy' which consists of 'producing large numbers of offspring and devoting relatively little attention to them' (a strategy adopted 'in general, [by] fish, reptiles and amphibia'). Caucasian and Mongoloid men, on the other hand, adopt a 'K strategy' that 'consists of producing few offspring and investing considerable energy in raising them' (a more mammalian strategy) (Lynn 1990: 1203). Thus Lynn enlists hormones to reproduce the well-worn racist argument that black men are lower forms of life than white men, while at the same time positioning Asian men as less masculine than white men.[26] The action of such racist discourses within the development of HRT for men is not yet as clear as it is for women, but it is, of course, most likely that HRT will be developed principally for wealthy men in the west. Arguments about racially differentiated hormonal levels may provide a resource for those needing to justify this practice.

Elixirs of difference

Hormones in the form of HRT message narrow versions of sexual, class and racial differences. This is evident in the logics of discourses promoting HRT use only for particular people.[27] These discourses facilitate the

---

[26] For other examples see Gould 1993; Stepan 1993. Haraway (1997: 204–5) analyses similar racist arguments about reproductive strategies.

[27] This targeted promotion of HRT to particular groups is successful. HRT is used disproportionately in wealthy western countries, such as the USA, Australia and Finland and is used much less in South East Asia, for example (European HRT–Network Foundation 2001). There is substantial evidence that women who take HRT in the USA are likely to be white, educated and reasonably well off (cited in Gullette 1997: 191; see also Avis *et al.* 2001: 350); 80 per cent of the women in the US-based Women's Health Initiative trial were 'white Caucasians' (Lam *et al.* 2005: 250). The first British study of ethnic differences in the use of HRT found that 'women from ethnic minority groups were less likely than white women to use hormone-replacement therapy' and that these differences were independent

production of two types of bodies: the 'natural' bodies of non-western people who do not need HRT and the 'unnatural' bodies of westerners who require hormonal supplementation in later life. These racialised representations of aging are connected to conventional figurations of sexual difference. In HRT discourses, hormones provide pleasantness and beauty to certain women and strength and penetrative ability to certain men. The provision is figured as a restoration of 'natural' differences disturbed by aging.

The promotion of HRT to 'restore' sexual differences takes place within an ongoing reconfiguration of western societies along bio-social lines. Most analyses of these changes focus on genetics and reproduction, arguing that the new genetics and reproductive technologies produce new forms of relationality and embodiment for those engaged with them (either directly or indirectly).[28] The case of HRT, as I have demonstrated here, has a longer history and is perhaps not as innovative a medical technology, but nonetheless resonates in terms of scale (the sheer numbers of HRT consumers) and also in terms of the ways in which HRT-taking becomes a medical supplement to everyday life in an ongoing manner (it is recommended that aging people take HRT for many years). What becomes clear in the case of HRT that is sometimes overlooked in the case of genetics is the centrality of sexual difference to bio-sociality.[29] A critical analysis of HRT discourses demonstrates that contemporary forms of bio-social subjectification are intimately tied to persistent figurations of sexual difference as binary, which are themselves linked to hierarchical understandings of racial differences. As this chapter has shown, discourses involved in the development, promotion and prescription of HRT actively reproduce sexed embodiments along racialised and classed lines. Sex hormones in the form of HRT, in other words, 'message sex' in aging bodies, producing a distinctively gendered form of bio-sociality deeply intertwined with economic considerations of markets and profits.

The analysis undertaken in earlier chapters suggested that hormones could be understood as active not only at discursive levels, but also in material, lived bodies – indeed, that hormones' messaging works 'across'

---

of smoking, age or hysterectomy (Harris *et al.* 1999: 610). The article does not attempt to provide any explanation for these differences.

[28] See, for example, Edwards *et al.* 1999; Rapp 1999; Finkler 2000; Franklin and Mackinnon 2003; Roberts and Franklin 2005; Franklin and Roberts 2006.

[29] Some feminist work on reproduction and the new genetics deals with these issues: see, for example, Rapp 1999; Rapp *et al.* 2001.

and therefore problematises, any distinction between the biological and the social. The argument in this chapter suggests that hormones are active within HRT discourses, both medical and popular. Chapter 5 moves this argument forward through an analysis of what hormones in the form of HRT actually do within bodies. How are HRT's messaging actions evident in bodies and how are they (inter)implicated in the production of material sexual differences?

5

The messaging effects of HRT

In her comparative analysis of menopause discourses in Japan and North America, anthropologist Margaret Lock suggests that aging women present a problem to contemporary societies. As discussed in Chapter 4, their very existence confounds enduring figurations of sexual difference as both binary and based on reproductivity. Women's move beyond (hetero) sexual exchange and reproduction challenges cultural conceptions of life itself. 'Women have a better survival rate than men', Lock writes,

> this cannot be denied, but the very fact that they live longer seems to count as a stroke against them. Elderly women can only be troublesome to society, it seems, as though the present average life expectancy for men is the way things should be, and anything more is unnecessary, especially if these women can contribute neither to the continuity of the species nor to the pleasure of men.
> *(Lock 1993: 365–6)*

For over forty years, hormone-replacement therapy (HRT) has been offered as a solution to this problem. HRT promises to alleviate the physical and psychological suffering of women going through menopause and, as far as possible, to maintain women's participation in circuits of sexual exchange. Medical claims about HRT, however, do not only refer to women's sexuality, appearance, temperament and reproductivity, they also focus on illness and disease. HRT has been said to play a role in the prevention of serious health problems associated with aging, namely, osteoporosis, heart disease, Alzheimer's disease, colon cancer and rheumatoid arthritis. This chapter focuses on these claims, analysing how they are mobilised in medical, pharmaceutical and health promotion discourses aimed at helping women to make decisions about whether or not to take HRT. Analysis of these discourses provides evidence of a contemporary trend in western biomedicine in which patients are reconfigured as active, informed decision-makers rather than passive recipients of medical care and pharmaceutical products. Working through the example of HRT, I critically investigate this reconfiguration and ask how it might be challenged by conceptualising hormones as active messengers of sex.

Intended effects and 'side' effects

Discussing the period of the mid-1920s, Nelly Oudshoorn states that 'Sex hormones could best be described as drugs looking for a market' (Oudshoorn 1994: 108). Although in the late twentieth century sex hormones in the form of HRT certainly secured a market, they might still be described today as drugs looking for a disease. For the debate about what *exactly* HRT does continued throughout the 1990s, with many claims about HRT's preventive effects being challenged in the early twenty-first century. In the period from the 1960s, HRT began as a miraculous antidote to aging, became an accepted and widely used medication and is now perceived, by its critics at least, as seriously flawed. In media controversies around the premature termination of the world's largest clinical trial of HRT in May 2002 (The Women's Health Initiative study) and the publication of the results of Britain's 'Million Women Study' in August 2003, statements about HRT became more negative than ever before. The *Guardian*'s front-page headline reporting the Million Women Study results states starkly, for example, that 'HRT treatment doubles risk of breast cancer' (Meikle 2003: 1). Commenting on these results two months later on the front page of the *Independent*, the chair of the German Commission on the Safety of Medicines, Professor Bruno Muller-Örlinghausen, describes HRT as 'the new thalidomide' and as a 'national and international tragedy', causing thousands of deaths (Laurance 2003: 1). The title of well-known American health activist Barbara Seaman's (2003) popular book, *The Greatest Experiment Ever Performed on Women: Exploding the Oestrogen Myth*, also evokes a sense of betrayal and reckless experimentation with women's bodies. How did these changes occur? And what are their implications for thinking about hormones as messengers of sex?

In the 1960s, HRT was described as an antidote to women's loss of 'femininity' (McCrea 1983; Bell 1987). In this period and up to the 1980s, HRT was marketed mainly as a treatment for menopausal symptoms such as hot flushes, atrophic vaginal changes and decreases in well being (Mitteness 1983). The ability to enjoy heterosexual intercourse and to maintain an emotionally supportive and happy attitude within heterosexual marriage was figured as an important outcome of HRT-taking. Sandra Coney (1991) analyses a set of pharmaceutical advertisements for HRT from this period, demonstrating the ways in which heteronormative femininity is linked visually and textually to HRT-taking (see also Palmund 1997). Some more recent advertisements for HRT, published in medical journals, continue to make such links. A 1993 Novo Nordisk advertisement for Trisquens® ('Complete HRT with just one tablet a day'), for example, depicts a middle-aged woman wearing pearls bursting joyfully from a worried and unhappy large-scale plaster model of her own head (Novo Nordisk 1993). Cilag's advertisments from the same period promise 'Emancipation!' and 'Liberation *for* women!' through HRT-taking (Cilag 1995, 1996, emphasis in original). Sepia-toned images of women dressed as defiant nineteenth-century suffragists chained to fences clarify this unnerving theme: rather than feminist politics, what offers women 'liberation' is an HRT patch that promises 'freedom from tablet taking' and 'release from symptoms of menopause'. Aging female biology is positioned here as oppressive – something that, with HRT consumption, can be thrown off. Through the co-option of political language and imagery, the advertisements imply that HRT will also liberate women from feminist politics. Unlike the depicted angry and pained activists obsessed with political suffrage, the woman taking Evorel® will be part of 'a new generation' who will cast 'a vote of confidence for HRT'. Her actions, in other words, will be directed towards her own body rather than to the public sphere or to her political rights.[1]

Alongside these claims that HRT will reduce menopausal symptoms and render women more pleasant and feminine, the 1990s medical literature and pharmaceutical campaigns cited a much wider range of conditions as being positively affected by HRT. The most important of these were osteoporosis and heart disease. These additional claims were also linked with substantial increases in numbers of women taking HRT; in the mid-1990s around 40% of target populations in countries like Australia

---

[1] The image of HRT as liberation has been long been part of popular HRT discourses. In his Foreword to Robert A. Wilson's *Feminine Forever*, Professor of Endocrinology Robert B. Greenblatt wrote that 'Woman will be emancipated only when the shackles of hormonal deprivation are loosed. Then, she will be capable of obtaining fulfilment without interrupting her quest for a continuum of physical and mental health' (Greenblatt, in Wilson 1966: 13). Wilson also uses the language of emancipation, but refers to sexual rather than feminist liberation, opening his book by describing women taking HRT as 'spearheading a new kind of sexual revolution' (Wilson 1966: 15). Wilson was no supporter of 1960s-style sexual liberation, however. Indeed, some pages on he writes, 'I am often disturbed at the blatancy with which women themselves proclaim their sexual liberation' (Wilson 1966: 25). HRT, for Wilson, was to preserve the kind of femininity that he, 'speaking as a male', preferred (Wilson 1966: 26).

and the USA had taken HRT at some time.[2] By 1999, US annual hormone therapy prescriptions were at 90 million, representing approximately 15 million women (Hersh *et al.* 2004). By 2001, the American HRT industry was worth $2.75 billion (Seaman 2003: 228) and with direct-to-consumer marketing of pharmaceutical products then legal, HRT was advertised on national television. In one such commercial, described in more detail later, the bone loss associated with women's aging is the specific indicator mentioned for an unnamed HRT product (Wyeth n.d.). Aging supermodel, Lauren Hutton, talks about refusing to take HRT for 'hot flashes and night sweats at menopause', but convinced by her sudden bone loss, deciding a year later that it *was* worth taking. 'And I've been on it for years', she states to camera, beaming (Wyeth n.d.).[3]

Osteoporosis is a chronic condition characterised by cumulative decreases in bone mass. Medical arguments about the positive effects of HRT on osteoporosis have a particular trajectory that is reproduced time and again. The basic pattern is to establish a frightening and expensive crisis (a high incidence of osteoporosis-caused fractures) and then to present HRT as the way to prevent or stem this crisis. The final step is to extrapolate the need for HRT to every (western) woman through the figuring of every woman as a potential participant in the crisis. Excerpts from an article in *Clinics in Geriatric Medicine* (1993) demonstrate this flow of argument:

> Osteoporosis is epidemic in the United States, currently affecting 15 to 20 million individuals ...
> Hip fractures alone occur in about 240 000 women per year with a mortality of 40 000 annually and an associated cost of billions of dollars ...
> Estrogen therapy stabilizes the process of osteoporosis or prevents it from occurring ...
> Once estrogen levels fall, either at menopause or following cessation of estrogen therapy, there is accelerated loss of bone; therefore, for maximal effect, therapy should begin as soon after menopause as possible and be continued for an indefinite period of time.
>
> *(Speroff 1993: 37)*

Despite the frequent repetition of this argument in the medical and scientific literature, controversy remains regarding the specificities of oestrogen's effects on bone density. The exact mechanisms by which

---

[2] See, for example, Ellerington, Whitcroft and Whitehead 1992: 422; Oddens *et al.* 1992; Worcester and Whatley 1992: 4; Dennerstein 1993/4: 12; Utian and Schiff 1994; Topo *et al.* 1995.

[3] Many thanks to Joseph Dumit for sending me videotaped examples of direct-to-consumer pharmaceutical advertisements. For more on this form of advertising, see Dumit 2005.

oestrogens affect bone density are not known – indeed it is not clear whether the effects are direct or indirect – and the effects of progestogens are even less clear (Prevelic and Jacobs 1997: 326). Importantly, arguments are also made in the medical literature against the automatic correlations drawn between bone density and fracture rates, based on the fact that other factors such as improved vision, mobility, balance and muscular strength have significant beneficial impacts on fall and fracture rates.[4]

In relation to bone mass, the effects of oestrogen are complicated by timing and duration of treatment, because whenever HRT is stopped, bone loss resumes or even accelerates (Johnston, cited in Klein and Dumble 1994: 336). In other words, HRT is thought only to stall bone loss, not ultimately to prevent it. In a review article on the menopause and post-menopause, Prevelic and Jacobs (1997) argue that oestrogen-only HRT (ERT) has a positive effect on bone density only for a certain period after treatment. ERT taken for 5–10 years from the beginning of menopause, for example, has little or no effect on bone loss or fracture risk at age 70, when fractures are most common (Prevelic and Jacobs 1997: 324). Taking ERT from the age of 65 may reduce fractures in the woman's late 70s and 80s, although the positive effects are seen to be less at this age. Given these factors, it has been suggested by some researchers that women should take HRT from menopause until death to avoid bone density deterioration. However, given that breast cancer risk increases with HRT use, this recommendation is troubling.[5] In 1998, Ettinger wrote, '[I]f women follow current recommendations for lifelong ERT use, their ultimate risk of breast cancer could double' (Ettinger 1998: 4).

Until 2002, HRT's 'protective' effects regarding heart disease were less controversial, although the mechanisms by which oestrogens prevent heart disease were unknown (Subbiah 1998; Luckas *et al.* 1998). Risk of heart disease was said by some to be halved by oestrogen-replacement therapy use, although this was disputed (Ettinger 1998: 3; Subbiah 1998: 24). In 2002, however, the world's largest randomised controlled trial of HRT, undertaken in the United States, was prematurely halted. This trial, which involved 16,500 women, demonstrated that rather than having a protective impact on heart disease risk, HRT-taking *increased* women's risk of this illness. It was concluded in the early part of this study that HRT 'should

---

[4] See Capezuti *et al.* 1998; Cobbs and Ralapati 1998: 140; Shaw and Snow 1998.

[5] See Brinton and Schairer 1993; Speroff 1993: 46–50; Adami and Persson 1995; Davidson 1995; Stanford *et al.* 1995; Prevelic and Jacobs 1997: 329–30; Zumoff 1998; Beral and Million Women Study Collaborators 2003.

not be initiated or continued for primary prevention of CHD [coronary heart disease]' (Writing Group for the Women's Health Initiative Randomized Controlled Trial 2002: 2). The authors also found that HRT increased the risk of invasive breast cancer and indeed this was the main reason the trial was halted. Summarising, the authors of the study concluded that 'overall health risks exceeded benefits from use of combined oestrogen plus progestin for an average 5.2-year follow-up among healthy postmenopausal US women' (Writing Group for the Women's Health Initiative Randomized Controlled Trial 2002: 2).

More contested claims have recently been made for HRT's effects on the brain. Whilst some argue that HRT improves performance on selected mental tasks within controlled studies (Sherwin 1998), others produce contrary evidence (Polo-Kantola et al. 1998). Some studies regarding the effects of HRT on women at risk of Alzheimer's disease or other dementias do not provide evidence of a positive effect (Yaffe et al. 1998), whilst others claim that HRT improves symptoms of dementia (Ettinger 1998: 3; Prevelic and Jacobs 1997: 326–8). The effects of HRT on women not at risk of dementia and on 'non-demented' women also remain in question (Yaffe et al. 1998; Polo-Kantola et al. 1998).

It is clear, then, that the effects of HRT are at once significant and contested. New indications are produced and investigated before older indications are substantiated. The emphasis on Alzheimer's disease and dementia, for example, is relatively new. Other new indications for HRT include colon cancer (Prevelic and Jacobs 1997), rheumatoid arthritis and diabetes (Adami and Persson 1995). There are also complicated questions concerning HRT's 'side' effects, especially cancer.[6] Although a number of studies in the 1990s found links between HRT use and increased risks of specific cancers (endometrial and breast cancer), others argued that these risks could either be avoided through the addition of progestogens to HRT in the case of endometrial cancer, or were not sufficiently substantial to argue against HRT use.[7] The largest British study of HRT, the Million Women Study, published in 2003, however, found that taking combined HRT for as short a period as 1–2 years does increase women's risk of breast cancer. Reported on the front page of leading British newspapers, the

---

[6] The concept of side effects is contentious; the use of 'side' to characterise unwanted or negative effects tends to minimalise their importance and to imply that drugs work in more targeted ways than they actually do.

[7] See Speroff 1993: 45–50; Adami and Persson 1995; Davidson 1995; Stanford et al. 1995; Prevelic and Jacobs 1997: 329–32; Zumoff 1998; Beral and Million Women Study Collaborators 2003.

study's results showed that 'the risks associated with the combined oestrogen-progestogen HRT are far higher than previously thought and begin much earlier than doctors assumed' (Frith 2003: 1). Read in conjunction with the premature termination of the Women's Health Initiative Trial, this study has created strong (yet still contested) doubts around the health benefits and risks of HRT-taking.

Biomedicine's response to the complexities of HRT's effects and the compelling yet contested evidence around these effects is twofold. Firstly and most commonly, reference is made to the individuality of the woman patient and to her personal responsibility in making decisions regarding HRT. This individualising emphasis will be discussed in the last part of this chapter. Secondly, reference is made to 'ideal oestrogens' (Subbiah 1998: 27): a desired medication that will have all the beneficial effects of HRT but fewer of the 'side' effects. The same is true for progestogens. As one research group writes, '[T]he search continues for new oral progestogens which are more "metabolically friendly" than those in current use' (Ellerington *et al.* 1992: 401). Hopes are stated that such hormones will be produced in the future: 'The future of ERT is bright', Ettinger wrote in 1998, 'The challenge of the 21st century is to determine the optimal HRT regime' (Ettinger 1998: 4). Remaining, as it does, within a narrow paradigm of treating menopause and aging-related conditions with sex hormones, this is an inadequate response to the issues raised regarding the complexities of the effects of HRT on women's bodies, but it is surprisingly common. An article from *Clinics in Geriatric Medicine* provides a further example, which shows the emphatic nature of such recommendations:

> Hormone therapy *should* be offered to most women as they consider their paths for successful aging. However, as for any pharmacological intervention, the benefits of treatment must outweigh the risk. The available data would appear to indicate that, for most women, this is in fact the case with current research into future hormonal therapies aimed at further improving the benefit risk ratio.
>
> *(Speroff 1997: 3, emphasis added)*

The function of such positive future projections is to maintain faith in 'progress' around HRT and to draw distinctions between the 'side' effects of the medications and their intended effects. Such projections allow for a continuing positive assessment of HRT, despite negative results from studies of its effects. Even after the potentially devastating results of the US and British large-scale trials, such hopes continue to emerge in the mainstream press. In December 2005, for example, the *Guardian* reported a scientist arguing on the basis of animal research that women should take HRT five to ten years *before* the menopause, as well as after it (Meikle 2005: 9).

Feminist responses to HRT

Feminist writers have most frequently reacted negatively to the continuing flow of claims regarding HRT. One common (radical feminist) response is to argue that underneath all these claims is an oppressive and misogynous attempt to control aging women. Germaine Greer's *The Change* (1991) and Sandra Coney's *The Menopause Industry* (1991) are two important examples. In both books, the authors stress the 'natural' status of menopause, in contrast to medicine's deficiency disease model. Long-term hormone-replacement medication is presented as one element of an increasing medicalisation of western women's lives, itself part of maintaining oppressive patriarchal societies. Both Greer and Coney encourage resistance to a model that describes all aging women as sick, vulnerable and decaying. They posit alternative representations of aging women as wise and powerful, enjoying a new phase of life beyond some of the cultural and physical limitations of being a woman in her reproductive years. Feminist critics such as these argue that rather than reducing aging women's problems to biological factors, cultural reasons for women's suffering should be examined and changed – a task, that as Greer writes, is beyond the expertise of doctors and must be taken on more broadly:

> The medicalization of the menopause is the last phase in the process of turning all the elements of female personality that do not relate to the adult male into pathology. Virginity is pathology; lack of interest in heterosexual intercourse on demand is pathology; 'excessive' involvement in mothering is pathology; middle-aged truculence and recalcitrance are the most pathological of all. Now we have pills for all of them and women are obediently taking them. Doctors cannot change social, cultural, economic or political conditions; they can only try to tailor the patient to fit better into her circumstances.
>
> *(Greer 1991: 138)*

The radical feminist approach to menopause privileges 'natural' bodily integrity and the absence of technological interventions. Australian scholars Renate Klein and Lynette J. Dumble, for example, link HRT to other reproductive technologies, such as IVF, arguing that all of these technologies demonstrate an attempt on the behalf of masculinist ('Rambo') gynaecologists to control women's bodies: 'We perceive HRT as interfering with a woman's bodily integrity similar to reproductive technologies at large' (Klein and Dumble 1994: 339). Like Barbara Seaman, Klein and Dumble refer to the prescription of HRT as a form of 'hit and miss experimentation with healthy mid-life women' (Klein and Dumble 1994: 339).

Although perhaps not dissenting from some of the implications of these strong critiques, feminists from other theoretical 'camps' contest the basis of these radical feminist claims, arguing that the appeal to 'natural' aging is unproductive and in fact reinforces the nature/culture split on which the medical model also rests.[8] Jennifer Harding (1997: 140), for example, argues that many feminist discussions of menopause position women along a continuum of 'empowerment' that lies between the two extreme positions of passive victim ('sick, misinformed, over-dependent on medicalisations and disempowered') and active feminist ('well, informed, engaging in non-medical and self-help practices and empowered'). This model suggests that women progress along this continuum as they gain access to knowledge. Harding is critical of this model for good reasons, arguing that it cannot acknowledge different women's abilities to gain access to particular forms of knowledge. Furthermore, this model 'produces the postmenopausal woman as a passive recipient of knowledge' (Harding 1997: 140). Rather than a political or interested discourse that participates in the production of bodies themselves, knowledge is understood as existing outside of power relations and is seen as something that can be used as a tool to liberate the oppressed. In this education model, Harding argues, feminist suggestions regarding menopause line up with medical models in so far as both rely on a separation between the body (understood as biology or 'nature') and knowledge (understood as 'culture').

Whilst Harding's critique is powerful, it is limited in regard to the resources it provides for thinking both about what HRT does in bodies and about how women can come to decisions regarding HRT. For although Harding is critical of an education model, her own approach seems ultimately to offer an even more complex version of knowledge promotion as the best avenue for women's decision-making regarding HRT. According to Harding, women must not only understand the medical aspects of HRT, they must become aware of the historically and socially constructed nature of HRT and biomedicine in general and be able to apply deconstructive thinking to their own lives. There is still a sense here of a valorised feminist position from which informed and correct decisions could be made about HRT. This position is achieved with extensive *feminist* knowledge.

What underlies both these forms of argument, then – the radical feminist position that sees HRT-taking as a form of oppression of naïve women and the poststructuralist position that promotes women's active and critical engagement with biomedicine, rather than refusal of it – is the desire for *an answer* to the question of HRT's effect on bodies. Given

---

[8] See Leysen 1996; Lupton 1996; Van Wingerden 1996; Harding 1997; Kwok 1997.

the complexities of bodies and of the 'working' of hormones within them, this desire is highly problematic. If we understand hormones as material-semiotic actors that message across – and thus disrupt any fixed distinctions between 'nature' and 'culture' – the reasons for this become clearer. As messengers, the hormones in HRT do not act (either discursively or materially) outside of specific bodily and cultural configurations. This is not to deny the existence of strong patterns of action that are repeated across different women's bodies, or across different historical or geographic domains, but rather to argue that the desire for a singular truth of HRT's effects will always be frustrated. The desire for such a truth by definition involves abstraction from the specificities of hormones' messaging actions in any particular instance, which is, if we understand hormones as active messengers within specific configurations of bodies, times and places, impossible. But where does this conceptualisation of hormones leave menopausal women trying to make decisions around HRT-taking? Does it mean that nothing meaningful can be said about the effects of hormones in bodies outside of individual cases?

Individual women's decisions: making medical choices

The absolute risk of harm to an individual woman is very small.
(Fletcher and Colditz 2002: 3)[9]

Contemporary medical science is unable to provide coherent or uncontested evidence regarding the risks and benefits of HRT for menopausal women. In acknowledging this problem, medical scientists gesture towards hopeful futures and more perfect drugs but also, 'in the meantime' (as if there will be a time in which 'the facts' are indisputable), place the burden of responsibility on individual women to make decisions about which medications they want to take. This movement of responsibility onto individual women resonates to some extent with the feminist literature on women's medical decision-making, but like all liberal models of 'choice' is cleansed of any engagement with issues relating to power differences. Women in these discourses are expected to be active in their choices of medication, but are 'liberated' in a way that has more to do with the 'freedom' represented in the Evorel® advertisement discussed earlier than with political change. This is change at the personal, biological level, isolated from public sphere or collective engagement. As I will

[9] Cited in Rayner 2002: 2 and Burkeman 2002: 2.

show, whether or not to take HRT becomes an almost impossible decision, one that, as recent empirical evidence demonstrates, is often removed from women in actual clinical encounters. Discourses of HRT-related choice operate strongly at a rhetorical level and contribute to the production of individual health-related responsibilities, without substantially challenging women's relation to their bodies, to femininity, or to medical authority.

Like some feminist arguments and media representations of the HRT debate, medical texts have high expectations of women when it comes to learning about HRT. An article from the *New England Journal of Medicine*, revealingly entitled (as if such a choice could be made), 'Hormone-Replacement Therapy: Breast versus Heart versus Bone', provides an excellent example. The author, Nancy E. Davidson, writes:

> Given our fragmented knowledge of therapy with estrogen alone or with estrogen plus a progestin, a prospective assessment of the net health effects of postmenopausal hormone therapy is badly needed … In the meantime, all postmenopausal women should be apprised of our current understanding of the risks and benefits of hormone-replacement therapy. They should pay particular attention to their own risk factors and the relative impact of cardiovascular disease, osteoporotic fractures, and cancer of the breast, colon, and uterus on women's health in general.
>
> *(Davidson 1995: 1639)*

The slippage in this quote from the discussion of 'our fragmented knowledge' and 'our current understanding' to the decision that women ('they') must make, 'pay[ing] particular attention to their own risk factors' and to the impact of particular, widespread diseases on 'women's health in general' is striking. Clearly 'we' are not menopausal women and are responsible only for objective knowledge. 'They' must calculate their own risks. And not only this, 'they' must do so with a view to choosing which diseases have the worst effects on 'women's health in general'. This is no light expectation.[10]

What is clear here is that each woman is expected to make medical decisions based not only on her own history, including her genetic

---

[10] This approach has only developed in recent years. Compare, for example, an affidavit used in the 1977 Pharmaceutical Manufacturers' Association's suit against the FDA's demand that oestrogen pill packages should include a warning insert: '[T]he insert will "interfere with the doctor–patient relationship, destroy a patient's trust in her physician and increase self-diagnosis and self-medication"' (Kaufert 1982: 157. Kaufert takes this quote from a 1977 health guide produced by the National Women's Health Network). Similarly, a 1980 article in *Current Therapy* argued that '[A] patient who has been frightened by "magazine articles" or "Food and Drug Administration bulletins" may "psychologically block the benefits" of ERT' (McCrea 1983: 117. McCrea quotes from an article by Kantor in *Current Therapy*).

inheritance ('Did your mother, grandmother or aunts have breast cancer, osteoporosis, heart disease ...?') but also to calculate the relevance of statistical knowledge to this history. From the myriad lives constituting statistical evidence of the effects of HRT, the menopausal woman contemplating taking HRT must discern which cases are relevant to her. She must do this not only in relation to her past and the past of her family, but also must project into the future and decide which diseases are more likely to happen to her, or which she most wants to avoid. This is the choice of Breast versus Heart versus Bone. As an article in the *International Journal of Fertility and Women's Medicine* states, 'The final decision to use therapy should be made by the patient, guided by her physician, and based on her current symptoms and her relative likelihood of developing coronary artery disease, osteoporotic fractures and cancer' (Hillard 1997: 347). Such choice can become quite absurd; anthropologist Emily Martin writes, 'One woman I talked to said her doctor gave her two choices for treatment of her menopause: she could take oestrogen and get cancer or she could not take it and have her bones dissolve' (Martin 1997: 246).

Such decisions can never be made on purely scientific, medical or rational grounds. An individual woman will not be able to find an exact model for herself in existing medical studies: someone who has lived the same number of years since menopause; who has or does not have 'an intact uterus'; who shares the exact risk factors for various diseases and the exact lifestyle factors regarding whether she smokes, drinks, works, lives in a middle-class suburb;[11] who belongs to the identical racial or ethnic group or, if a migrant, has lived in the new country for the same length of time[12] and so on. The singularity of any woman's experience cannot be replicated in statistical studies. Despite this, women are expected to undertake assessments of their own situations and make informed decisions.

A recent leaflet produced by Trisquens® manufacturer Novo Nordisk, entitled 'Choosing HRT: weighing up the facts', provides an example of how this imperative works in practice (Novo Nordisk n.d.). Produced in the aftermath of the premature termination of the Women's Health Initiative Trial and the results of the Million Women study, this scientific-looking side of A4 (no pictures, a graph and lots of text) makes only a weak

---

[11] US studies demonstrate that working-class women who live in working-class neighbourhoods are more likely to have high blood pressure than working-class women who live in more affluent neighbourhoods (Krieger and Fee 1996: 26).

[12] Australian statistics show that the incidence of certain diseases in particular ethnic groups is closer to a national norm for immigrants who have lived longer in the new country (Madden 1994).

assertion that it might be helpful to women, stating that 'This leaflet has been produced to help you decide whether HRT is right for you. Weighing up the associated benefits and potential risks *may* help you to make that decision (Novo Nordisk n.d., emphasis added). Listing the '*associated* benefits' first, the leaflet makes strong claims without any statistical evidence, including both the relief of menopausal symptoms and the prevention of osteoporosis and coronary heart disease as the outcomes of taking HRT. Moving on to the '*potential* risks', however, the leaflet moves into the realm of statistics. (Arguably, this use of statistics produces the risks as more contentious than the benefits, which require no statistical or graphical evidence, but are simply stated as 'facts'.) 'You may be concerned about the possibility of developing breast cancer while on HRT', the leaflet asserts (and if the reader has kept up with the media coverage of the HRT trials, this is indeed highly likely and rational). Stating the logical truism that 'All women are at risk of developing breast cancer, whether they are on HRT or not', the leaflet then runs its deceptively simple statistical argument. Using a basic bar graph, the reader is shown how the number of women 'likely to be diagnosed with breast cancer' increases with the length of time they have taken HRT. This statistical fact is explained as if it correlates with a specific (and very small) number of women. 'For women aged fifty who start HRT', the leaflet argues, 'only an extra 6 in 1,000 cases will be diagnosed after 10 years.' 'Only 6 women', the reader could be forgiven for thinking, 'that's not very many.' We are not told how many women this refers to in any one year, or told which women these might be; in contra-distinction to the emphasis on individuality and the specificity of particular experiences of menopause evident in many medical and self-help publications, 'women' here constitute an undifferentiated category. The leaflet also provides statistics on 'the risk of developing deep vein thrombosis, 3 in 10,000 whilst taking HRT, in comparison to 1 in 10,000 for women not taking HRT'. Again, no information is given as to who these women might be or what the significance or meaning of these statistics is. These statistics are described in small print at the bottom of the page as 'some of the necessary facts required to help you make a well-informed decision about HRT'. Without at least a working knowledge of statistics or epidemiology, however, these are meaningless numbers. Their function is to demonstrate that the risks associated with HRT are minimal and only 'potential', in contrast to the benefits, which are 'wide ranging'.

This leaflet demonstrates a cynical use of statistics to encourage women to make particular health decisions (to use this company's product). But are there other ways that statistics can function in decision-making? Statistics are a method of observation that attempts to render a state of affairs objective and factual, but, as Donna Haraway argues, 'Objectivity is less about realism than it is about intersubjectivity' (Haraway 1997: 199). Although Haraway uses this idea to make a point about the nature of scientific objectivity and to argue for the importance of good statistics to feminist projects around public health, this intersubjectivity of statistics might also be thought in a more intimate way. For the individual trying to decide whether or not to take HRT, statistics regarding menopause, the effects of these medications and the incidence of disease, could sharply bring home the point that this very personal experience – of aging, temperature, time, cell growth and bleeding – is a constructed and shared event, in which the bodies and lives of other, unknown women come to hold significant meaning in one's own life decisions. In this sense, statistics could produce the opposite effect to their scientifically situated position; rather than demonstrating the objective and detached nature of biology, they can show that experiences of the flesh are complex, situated and produced in particular sites across the globe at differing levels of intensity. A woman's experience of menopause is made intersubjective through the (attempted) application of statistics to her experience. The singularity of her experience can be realised through the lives of those represented in these numbers.

Within the medical literature, any woman considering taking HRT is asked to think about her life in terms both historical and predictive. In other words, the menopausal woman is expected to think of her present (her current decision) through the folding of her past (her genetic inheritance and the history of her body in illness and health) into her future (the likelihood of various diseases). Then she is asked to consider her life in relation to that of others – as an individual, the menopausal woman must think of 'the relative impact of cardiovascular disease, osteoporotic fractures, and cancer of the breast, colon, and uterus *on women's health in general*' and make decisions for herself in terms of this impact (Davidson 1995: 1639; emphasis added). The intersubjectivity of statistics thus folds the lives of other unknown women into the individual woman's experience.

In this model, medical decision-making becomes a process of applying mathematical calculations of risk to one's own life and thinking of hormones as complex biological actors with multiple potentialities for relieving and causing physical suffering. The intellectual work involved is demanding and can become, as Emily Martin's example shows, 'absurd'. Framed as 'choice', these decisions are represented in the mainstream press as a labour of selection. In 2002, for example, journalist Claire Rayner wrote of her own decision to take HRT in the *Guardian*, suggesting that women should decide whether they want the short-term benefits of symptom relief, or would prefer to live longer (by not, as she did, contracting breast cancer): 'Work out what you want or don't want', she advocates, 'Look at the facts regarding HRT (and, yes, this is the time to look at the science bit) and make your choices from there' (Rayner 2002: 3).

In pharmaceutical advertisements, patient literature and media articles (including websites), women are advised to seek help with such decision-making through discussions with general practitioners and in some cases are given lists of questions to stimulate appropriate discussions with doctors. A recent British Department of Health-sponsored patient leaflet, for example, offers the following list of prompts: 'Could HRT help me?' 'Does it cost anything?' 'Are there other options for treating my symptoms?' (Health Promotion England 2000: 17). In newspapers too, women are encouraged to speak to their doctors in making HRT-related decisions. In practice, however, women find it extremely difficult to follow this advice in interacting with clinicians. This is demonstrated in several recent studies showing that in medical clinics in England, Wales and Sweden, women are unable or highly reluctant to ask questions about HRT prescription (Hunter, O'Dea and Britten 1997; Elwyn *et al.* 1999; Henwood *et al.* 2003; Hoffman *et al.* 2005). In interviews after clinical consultations in a British study, for example, women reported that they did not want to upset the doctors by asking questions (Henwood *et al.* 2003). Empirical (observational, simulation and interview-based) studies of doctors also show that decisions to prescribe HRT are often made *before* discussion with patients and that doctors believe that it is right to persuade women to take this medication (Elwyn *et al.* 1999: 756; Murtagh and Hepworth 2003a; Hoffman *et al.* 2005). In all of these studies, notably, women left clinics with prescriptions for HRT, even if they did not want to take this medication.

Australian research also complicates the idealised story of women's involvement in complex decision-making represented in the medical literature, pharmaceutical campaigns and the media (Murtagh and Hepworth 2003a, 2003b). In her ethnographic study of five menopause clinics in Melbourne, science-studies theorist Marilys Guillemin (2000a, 2000b) articulates the multiple ways in which women's complex understanding of the bio-social nature of their problems around menopause is funnelled into a hormone deficiency model. Although initially going to clinics principally to get information, in attending public seminars, filling in self-report questionnaires and having clinical measurements (such as bone density) taken, women came to understand their wide-ranging problems as symptoms of oestrogen deficiency. Over a period of time women actively took on this biomedical model, so that when they finally met with a doctor to decide whether or not to take HRT, they were already participating in a way of thinking that leads 'inevitably' to hormone medication. One interviewee reported her experience of a lack of choice in relation to HRT prescription:

> I had gone to the menopause clinic wanting to get more information and I was virtually put straight on HRT, or after the first visit when I had tests and things. In a way I was a bit shocked because they seem to have taken it for granted that's what I wanted and didn't really tell me if there were any alternatives. But from what I've read I sort of felt that it probably was inevitable but they didn't seem to tell me of anything else that I might have done and not gone on to HRT. They just seemed to take it for granted that was to happen.
>
> *(in Guillemin 2000b: 19)*

This empirical evidence throws doubt on the existence of real opportunities for women to engage in serious dialogue with clinicians around HRT-related decision-making. In all of these studies, women leave clinical encounters with prescriptions for drugs they did not desire. The rhetoric around women's choice and the concept that, as the Wyeth television commercial puts it, 'HRT is not for all women', serves a different function to producing clinical spaces in which concerns around HRT can be seriously explored. This rhetoric does not translate into clinical practice (even in best-case scenarios, according to Hoffman and colleagues) but rather works to produce a certain instantiation of the HRT-taking woman (future *and* present, i.e. those who will take HRT and those who already do). These discourses produce a feminine subject who acts responsibly in engaging in almost impossible conceptual work around her body, but who in practice is usually deprived of acting on this work. Such a woman could be understood as an active consumer of biomedicine, but her activity, arguably, remains quite constrained. Contemporary women are expected to know more about their bodies and about the risks associated with medical treatments of menopausal symptoms, but this knowledge does not open up spaces of refusal or critique of biomedicine. The development of knowledge around the menopause does not create connections between women that could lead to political engagement, but rather configures women as engaged, active consumers of biomedical logics and products.

This use of knowledge to produce a particular kind of consumer is represented in the Wyeth television commercial for HRT mentioned earlier. In the opening shot, speaking to camera in a confessional mode, aging supermodel Lauren Hutton confides:

> When I started having hot flashes and night sweats at menopause, my doctor recommended hormone-replacement therapy, but I didn't listen. Up to 20% of a woman's expected lifetime bone loss occurs in the years following menopause. A year later I went back to my doctor and found I'd shrunk an inch! I went on HRT and I've been on it for years!
>
> *(Wyeth n.d.)*

Learning to 'listen' helps Hutton stall her bone loss and resultant 'shrinking' and to 'feel great'. A convert to engaged patienthood, she instructs her female audience to 'Talk to your doctor about the benefits and risks. The time to protect your future', she affirms, 'is now.' Although music from a women's choir swells up to complete the advertisement, female solidarity has not been represented here. Learning to listen and to talk to your doctor has one goal: to move you towards HRT.

HRT-taking women and bio-social embodiment

HRT discourses rhetorically figure HRT-taking women as active decision-makers and in practice produce them as valuable consumers of pharmaceutical products. I have argued above, however, that individual women's processes of decision-making about HRT *also* have the capacity to bring the profound complexity of human bodily experience, at least theoretically, to the fore. In asking women to weave a path through a complex set of folding processes in which an individual's experiences are positioned in relation not only to her own history and future but also to the experiences of others, medical HRT-related discourses open up space to refigure the actions of hormones. The configuration of the HRT-taking woman's body as situated in relation to the bodies of others (past, present and future) shows that bodily experience is never 'biological' in the sense of being outside of culture or non-relational, but rather involves the complex folding of history, culture and the experiences of others, *with* the biological.

But what does 'the biological' mean here? As discussed throughout this book, contemporary feminist theorists argue that human bodies are always historically and culturally produced and situated. This is in contrast to Enlightenment understandings of bodies, which position them as outside culture, as 'a timeless part of nature' (Gatens 1996: 66). Embodiment, then, involves a complex set of relations weaving between and among the biological and the social, continually (re)producing each body. The capacities and contents of bodies and biology are not predetermined but emerge and change through these relations. Cultural and psychical experiences are seen to be in interaction with the biological to produce what Gatens (1996) calls 'imaginary' and Grosz (1994) 'volatile' bodies. Grosz describes this interaction as a Möbius strip – an inverted figure eight – in which the biological and the social are figured as the two sides of the twisted figure. These two sides are neither identical nor radically disjoined but 'have the capacity to twist one into each other' (Grosz 1994: 209–10). Thus, as discussed in Chapter 3, the biological and the social are in constant and inseparable interrelation or 'interimplication' (Grosz 1994: 21).

It is central to these theories that embodiment is, to a large extent, culturally shared. Culturally prevalent sets of bio-social relations are embodied in all individuals, albeit to differing degrees. Thus history is important not only on an individual level – that person's life history – but creates embodiments across generations within and across cultures. Certain expectations of women's physical capacities, for example, are embodied by individuals and are shared across vast numbers of women, in part through their repetitive participation in certain physical actions which literally (re)produce particular bodies (Gatens 1996: 68–71). Understandings of the location or extension of various body elements are also culturally shared, in part through our use of language. Gatens (1996: 12) cites the example of hysterical paralysis of the arm, in which paralysis commonly ends where a sleeve would meet the shoulder seam rather than where physiology understands an arm to extend. This example demonstrates that most people in western cultures share a 'commonsense' understanding of arms that may be different from biomedical conceptions.

From this argument we could expect particular populations of menopausal women to share certain forms of embodiment in their aging. It is these embodiments that, as Guillemin's study showed, are funnelled into biomedical models through the practices of menopause clinics. If each woman had a unique experience of menopausal embodiment, this process would be impossible. Anthropological work provides interesting evidence of this point. Lock's comparison of the experiences of menopause in Japanese and North American women found that major symptoms of menopause are different in each country and indeed are symptoms that are infrequent in the other country. Hot flashes are considered a key symptom of menopause in the United States, but are rarely reported in Japan. Shoulder stiffness is not at all significant in the American menopause literature, but is a common complaint of Japanese women of menopausal age. As Lock (1993: 373) argues, these data demonstrate 'the plasticity of biology and its inter-dependence with culture'. Medical practices, then, must work with the prevalent embodiments in the culture they are operating within – a singular biomedical model could not be imposed with equivalent effect across different cultures (see, for example, Oudshoorn 1996b).

Conceptualising 'the biological', then, becomes complex; traditional understandings of the distinctions between the biological and the social, nature and culture are disrupted both by theoretical analyses and by anthropological studies. If, as Gatens, Grosz and Butler suggest, bodies are produced through repetitions of social actions and are inflected by psychical and shared cultural understandings, the lines between biology and the social must be constantly mobile. My argument throughout this book has been that hormones *message across this mobile boundary*, disrupting any attempts at delineating what belongs in each category, or indeed where the outline of the categories might lie. It is this mobility that is represented by the hyphen in 'bio-social'. In the case of HRT, the figuration of hormones as active messengers becomes quite concrete. Hormones in the form of HRT move into bodies in highly cultural, technical forms (patches, tablets, pessaries, creams) and do so within complex sets of discourses (biomedical, personal, economic, commercial). The bodies they move into are also culturally produced and situated. Thus HRT's effects cannot be separated from the complex interrelations between embodied experiences and the active world or 'nature'. Just as the side-effects of HRT cannot be isolated from its intended effects, its biological effects cannot be isolated from the historically and socially folded embodiments of those who take it.

Finally, even as biomedical technologies, hormones cannot be removed from the social into a purely technical or biological realm of activity. As messengers, sex hormones can be understood as actors involved in complex interactions: between entities within the body; scientists and laboratory entities used in experiments; historical and cultural understandings of sexual and other differences; and the situated experiences of particular bodies. Exogenous hormones, such as those in HRT, are also involved in additional interactions. They are actors in exchanges between a wide set of human and non-human actors, including: pharmaceutical companies and advertising agencies; general practitioners and patients; the pregnant mares whose urine is used to provide oestrogen and the technologies used in production and packaging; scientists experimenting with hormones and the journals that publish their work. Understood in this way, HRT's effects only happen within an ongoing and repetitive process of complicated interactions. It is impossible, I suggest, to separate out the biological from the social in these interactions.

In their narratives around hormones, however, the biomedical sciences *do* attempt to separate the effects of hormones (in the form of HRT, for example) from these complex interactions. Donna Haraway (1997: 68) would call this 'boundary-making and maintenance work' undertaken in order to keep 'stories and facts' at a 'respectable distance'. Building on the work of Bruno Latour, Oudshoorn (1996a) suggests that this striving for universal and decontexualised knowledge is one of the distinctive features of modern science and technology. This striving, Oudshoorn argues, results in a two-fold process:

> First, scientists create the contexts in which their knowledge claims are accepted as scientific facts and in which their technologies can work. Scientists adopt what I would call a '(re)contextualisation strategy' in which their knowledge claims gain momentum. Second, scientists then conceal the contexts from which scientific facts and artefacts arise, in a process which I will refer to as a 'decontexualisation strategy'.
>
> *(Oudshoorn 1996a: 124)*

These decontextualisation strategies are one of main avenues by which science produces its claim to objectively represent nature. In relation to medical technologies, such as HRT, this strategy of decontextualisation promises that any technology will 'work everywhere' or be universally applicable to individual users.

In the case of HRT, medical practitioners have to develop a decontextualisation strategy in the face of contradictory evidence about the effects of HRT. The knowledge claims associated with HRT remain uncertain and beyond quite general statements that, as a British National Health Service brochure (Health Promotion England 2000: 14) puts it, HRT can 'ease or prevent some of the uncomfortable symptoms associated with the menopause', there is much contestation. Even though medical practitioners conceal the contexts from which the scientific facts and artefacts constituting HRT arise, they cannot move claims about HRT's effects onto solid ground. Shifting responsibility for the complexities of these effects onto individual women patients, then, functions in a sense to paper over this deficit. HRT might not 'work' (have the desired symptom relief *and* preventive effects) for some women, but it will for others. As it is difficult for medical practitioners to say who these women will be, individuals must 'make their own decisions'.

This process of shifting responsibility produces a kind of decontextualisation: HRT is represented as simply 'doing what it says on the box' whilst the element of variability resides in individual women and their decisions about taking it. HRT in this sense is decontextualised through the contextualisation of women's differences from each other. My line of argument, however, suggests an alternative reading of HRT discourses: as a medical technology, HRT is designed to 'work' for some people and is situated within a set of clinical and cultural processes that functions to produce this group of 'configured users' of HRT-taking women.[13] The HRT-taking woman is the person represented in the medical literature and pharmaceutical advertisements and addressed by leaflets and television commercials as a thoughtful and active subject of contemporary biomedicine. She is the woman who, after engaging in a cost/benefit analysis, leaves the menopause clinic or general practitioner's office with a prescription for an HRT product. In this sense, one could argue, HRT is *not* decontextualised, but rather spreads its context onto the bodies of a (very large) group of women HRT-takers.

Bio-social messaging

Aging women make decisions about whether or not to take HRT within a complex scenario. Representations of HRT – in the popular press, in pharmaceutical advertisements and, anecdotally at least, in discussions amongst women – present two strong claims about HRT: its ability to address symptoms of menopause; and its efficacy in preventing long-term health problems. In the first case, narrow versions of sexed embodiment are reproduced: pictures of women smiling or of feminists 'freed' from the shackles of oestrogen-deficiency-induced politics suggest that taking HRT affirms a particular version of obliging femininity, 'contribut[ing] to the pleasure of men' (Lock 1993: 356). In regard to HRT's preventive capacities, significant contestations and differences in opinion abound. In reading leaflets and other medical literature, women are (at best) exposed to complex calculations of risk and benefit and are asked to take into account their individual and family pasts and futures, as well issues pertaining to 'women's health in general' (Davidson 1995: 1639). In medical consultations, however, these calculations are seemingly swept aside, as women become unheard participants in consultations in which GPs make

---

[13] The term 'configured user' was generated by Steve Woolgar (1993) and has been used by Oudshoorn (1996a), Madeleine Akrich (1992) and Susan Leigh Star (1991) amongst others, to describe the actors who designers imagine and 'build into' their technologies as they make them.

decisions, or are produced, through a series of staged engagements with menopause clinics, as inevitable consumers. Women exposed to radical feminist and other critical approaches to western medicine will also encounter powerful representations of menopause as part of a natural aging process that should be celebrated rather than treated or treated in alternative ways (with plant-based oestrogens such as phytosoya, or black cohosh, for example). All of these discourses produce the spaces of HRT-related decision-making as highly problematic.

It has been suggested here that the difficult terrain of such decision-making may be usefully reconfigured through a rethinking of the body and, indeed, of sex hormones themselves. Rather than being viewed as 'merely' biological entities, sex hormones within bodies (both endogenous hormones and HRT) might be thought of as material-semiotic or bio-social actors – as active participants in the production of particular, situated bodies. Like all human bodies, these situated bodies will be sexed/gendered. Hormones in the form of HRT are active in the production of heteronormative versions of sexed/gendered embodiments, but this does not happen only at the representational level. If hormones are thought of as bio-social actors, they can be understood as quite possibly active in the production of moods, cellular changes and feelings of desire within and between historically and geographically located bodies.[14] This action is not 'simply biological' in a traditional sense, however. Sex hormones in HRT co-act with representations of their actions, with social understandings of sex/gender, with lived embodied experiences and with specific processes of work, production and interaction between human and non-human actors. HRT-taking always occurs in articulation with representations of HRT's activity through the invocation of sexed/gendered norms, including the new norm of the active, engaged consumer of bio-medicine, which, as I will argue more fully in Chapter 6, is notably sexed/gendered. HRT is produced, prescribed and taken within networks of representation, interaction and already sexed/gendered bodies.

Today, menopausal women are put in an almost impossible position when making decisions about taking HRT. The considerations they are asked to make regarding their own histories, presents and futures are onerous. Placed next to empirical evidence about what actually happens when women engage with biomedical practitioners, this expectation of a high level of responsible and reflexive consideration appears absurd, as

---

[14] Cultural theorist Teresa Brennan (2004) makes an interesting argument about hormones and the transmission of affects and moods within groups.

women seem rarely able to make interventions into a process that assumes the prescription of HRT and does not provide meaningful alternatives. The radical feminist approach of outright resistance to medicalisation – of refusal to see menopause as a condition requiring treatment at all – is one response to this scenario.[15] Interestingly, the impact of the premature cessation of the Women's Health Initiative Trial indicates that such resistance is already occurring in relation to HRT. According to a study published in the *Journal of the American Medical Association*, after the announcement of the trial's unexpected findings US prescriptions of HRT in January–June 2003 declined by up to 66% (Hersh *et al.* 2004). If this trend continued, numbers of prescriptions should have returned to 1995 levels (57 million, rather than 90 million) by July 2003. North American women, then, are not becoming consumers of HRT in the numbers they did previously; once HRT's preventive message was challenged, it became a less attractive product.

Many social scientists, including feminists, have written about the reconfiguration of the consumer of contemporary biomedicine as an active, engaged individual, what Novas and Rose (2000) name 'the somatic individual'.[16] Although there are aspects of the history of this change that are strongly feminist and/or critical – the central role of women's health movements in changing women's relation to doctors and to their own bodies, or the importance of patient movements around HIV/AIDS, for example – these reconfigurations can be appropriated by biomedicine in problematic ways. The aim of feminist or gay/queer activism around health was neither simply to increase choice for individuals, nor to burden women or people living with HIV/AIDS with a set of impossible decisions. Likewise, in the case of HRT, it does not seem an adequate political response to the complexities of biomedical knowledge about hormones' effects on aging women's bodies to suggest that individual women educate themselves enough to make smart decisions. This education model places

---

[15] This sort of outright resistance to biomedical subjectifications is difficult to study empirically, as most social scientific researchers working on health recruit subjects via the subjects' engagement with biomedical institutions. In a fascinating case study from their broad-ranging research project on muscular dystrophy, French sociologists Michel Callon and Volona Rabeharisoa (2004) describe one man, Gino, who refuses all connection with biomedicine. They suggest that his refusal to attend medical consultations, to engage in the activities of patient activist and support groups, or to discuss genetic testing with his children, indicate a refusal of the subjectivity offered by contemporary biomedicine. Gino will not make choices from within a set offered to him by others or to explain his choices in the public sphere.

[16] See also Rabinow 1992; Rapp *et al.* 2001; Katz and Marshall 2003; Helén 2004.

untenable responsibility on individual women and, as Harding (1997) argued, ignores women's differing opportunities to develop knowledge. It also ignores the impossibility of choices offered (between different types of cancer, or between short- and long-term benefits, for example) and retains hope for 'the right answer' or singular truth about HRT's potential effects.

Moving away from the current ethical cul-de-sac in which biomedicine shifts untenable responsibilities onto women in the face of significant scientific and biological uncertainties requires a reconceptualisation of the very movement of hormones into bodies. Understanding the movement of hormones into bodies via HRT as a form of messaging across the shifting boundaries of the social and the biological provides a change of perspective. Hormones are no longer conceived as definitively knowable objects, but rather as actors involved in complex interactions with human and non-human actors. The bodies into which they move are never 'simply' biological, but are always situated, lived and sexed/gendered. The interactions between all the actors involved in HRT discourses, including representations of the HRT-taking woman, become political matters, requiring collective critical attention. Ultimately, then, questions about 'the paths to successful aging' should not be left up to individual women to 'consider' (Speroff 1997: 3), but rather must be framed and debated in a more public, political way. If HRT has been 'the greatest experiment ever performed on women', as Barbara Seaman claims, then we will need resources other than liberal conceptions of choice to challenge the discourses constituting it.

Materially, this shift requires serious change, including the development of new ways of talking about the menopause and HRT in patient literature, self-help books and websites and the creation of new forms of political engagement with regulators, governments, clinicians' representative bodies and pharmaceutical companies. Rhetorics of individual choice should be critiqued and resisted; we should not blame individuals for either prescribing or taking HRT, but rather work to configure new planes for consideration of such decisions that are not contained within individual life stories or clinical settings. Individual decisions will continue to need to be made in clinics, but they should not begin or end there. The biopolitics of hormones embodied in HRT are too significant for this.

I suggest that the responsibility for recommendations about the 'risks' of HRT-taking needs to be redistributed. It is not enough to repeat the mantra that risks are ultimately individual – these are risks that societies bear as much as individuals (if more women have cancer, we all suffer). We need more discussion of what the statistical risks mean to us as collectives and more open acknowledgement of which and whose interests are at stake in the prescription and taking of HRT. We need more and safer alternatives to preventing or treating the symptoms of menopause and preventing cancer in older women. Redistributing this responsibility does not mean that doctors should make decisions for women, however. I am not advocating a reaffirmation of paternalism in biomedicine! But decision-making needs to be disarticulated from responsibility and individuals understood as part of complex social formations of knowledges, practices and bodies. Whilst specific individuals must make decisions about patches, pills, phytosoya or black cohosh, these decisions should be figured, collected and analysed as part of broader enactments of contemporary sexed embodiment. Understanding our 'individual' decisions in this way – and figuring hormones as active in our engagements with them – undermines the absurd attribution of personal responsibility for idealised medical encounters and biological outcomes and creates space for more collective forms of (bio)-ethical or ethopolitical thought and practice.

6

Hormones in the world

Nobody can be sure whether environmental estrogens lie behind the
quadrupling of infertility rates since 1965; if the sea of estrogens in
which we live explains the fact that sperm counts are half of what they
were in 1940; and if, like intersex fish and mutant frogs, male humans
might begin to morph into women. Faced with the possibility of an all-
female planet, authorities might finally have to sidestep the pharmaceutical companies and take action.

(Seaman 2003: 222)

Globally today, a group of chemicals in the air and in water, food and
everyday household products, are suspected to be radically changing
human and non-human bio-social systems. Known as environmental oestrogens or endocrine-disrupting chemicals, these substances behave like
and/or disrupt endogenous sex hormones. Most of them are human-made
products of the twentieth century, deriving from both banned and everyday substances: plastics and phthalates (chemicals used to make plastics
flexible); pesticides such as DDT, dieldrin and chlordane; heavy metals like
lead, cadmium and mercury; perfumes and musks; flame retardants; cleaning products; and industrial chemicals and by-products such as PCBs
and dioxins. Endocrine disruptors exist in invisible, often infinitesimal,
quantities – they can be active in parts per trillion (Solomon and Schetter
2000: 1474) – and are found in every part of the globe. According to reports
from environmental non-governmental organisations like the World
Wildlife Fund for Nature (WWF 1999: 3), 'There is no clean, uncontami-
nated place anywhere on Earth and no creature untouched by this legacy.'

Endocrine disruptors engage in multiple activities: some act like hormones in the body, mimicking their actions and accentuating existing patterns, whilst others block the actions of endogenous hormones through
binding with hormone receptors and preventing usual effects. Still others

work in more complex ways, changing the actions of endogenous hormones and even genes. As well these differences of type, the effects of endocrine disruption are altered by the amount and timing of exposure to the toxicant: foetuses, for example, are understood to be especially vulnerable. As ubiquitous and indiscriminate actors, endocrine-disrupting chemicals disturb multiple boundaries: of time, generation, sex, geography and species. Stories of hormone-related devastation in scientific journals, environmental organisations' reports and the mass media – stories of rising infertility in men and women, of increasing incidence of reproductive cancers in humans, of reproductive system birth defects in children, of tiny penises in alligators, 'lesbian' seagulls and intersexed fish – elaborate these boundary crossings.[1] In these stories, both animals and humans are understood to be in profound danger, facing shared risks that indicate our conjoined lot of living in toxic, oestrogen-saturated environments; what health activist and writer Barbara Seaman, along with many others, calls a 'sea of oestrogens'.

Human reproductive health is a central concern in these stories. A recent review of the relevant scientific literature graphically depicts trends in reproductive health that may be affected by environmental oestrogens (Sharp and Irvine 2004: 449). These US figures show steep rises in rates of testicular and breast cancer and hypospadias (deformations of the penis) and significant decreases in sperm production. Sharpe and Irvine argue that these findings are well documented but that their causes – specifically their connection to endocrine disruptors – remain strongly contested:

> [I]t remains a topic of heated debate as to whether the potential of endocrine disruptors to disrupt hormone action and cause ill health in humans is a reality or merely a remote, theoretical possibility. What has fuelled this debate has been the increase in incidence of two hormone dependent disorders in humans over the last 70 or more years, namely breast cancer and testicular dysgenesis syndrome (comprising low sperm counts, testicular cancer, crytorchordism, and hypospadias).

> *(Sharpe and Irvine 2004: 448)*

Media reports, popular books and environmental campaigns also focus on decreasing sperm counts and increases in reproductive cancers and argue that foetuses and newborns have to struggle against their mother's hormonally toxic bodies.[2] Detailing the ways in which all of our bodies are

---

[1] See, for example, Raloff 1994a and 1994b; Stone 1994; World Wildlife Fund 1997 and 1998; National Research Council 1999; Lombardi *et al.* 2001; Sultan *et al.* 2001.

[2] See, for example, Raloff 1994b; Colborn *et al.* 1996: 173; Cadbury 1998: x; Riley, Bell and Warhurst 1999; World Wildlife Fund 1999; Berkson 2000; Friends of the Earth 2001c; Lombardi *et al.* 2001.

saturated with human-made chemicals, these reports (and related awareness-raising campaigns) advise women to breastfeed their babies but warn that this process leaches toxic chemicals out of women's bodies into the more vulnerable young.[3] Giving information about the dangers of household and personal products – cleaning fluids, perfumes, cosmetics and chemicals in furnishings, carpets and food – these discourses produce new responsibilities for women to protect future generations from the insidious effects of 'hormonally active' environments, including their own bodies.

The extent of this emerging discourse indicates that endocrine disruption has become a key site in which sex hormones actively message across the shifting and unclear boundaries of nature and culture today. Claims about endocrine-disrupting chemicals require sustained attention: the changes that they are said to stimulate raise significant health and environmental concerns. However, in taking these claims seriously it is also important to analyse the language used to describe sex hormones and their impact on bodies, behaviours and sexual difference. Seaman, for example, claims that 'male humans might begin to morph into women' and that authorities are 'faced with the possibility of an all-female planet' (Seaman 2003: 222). What is at stake in these powerful and provocative claims about biological sex and reproduction? What are the assumptions about the role of hormones inherent here? In this chapter, I critically analyse a range of discourses around environmental oestrogens, examining the ways in which they both problematically mobilise historical understandings of the actions of sex hormones *and* challenge mainstream scientific conceptions of the hormonally sexed body. I ask how feminists might critically approach these discourses and take the messaging actions of environmental oestrogens seriously, without recourse to heteronormative understandings of sexed biologies.

Describing 'gender-bending' chemicals

Popular scientific, mass media and environmentalist descriptions of what journalist Janet Raloff (1994a) calls 'the gender benders' mobilise two key material-semiotic histories: one relating to technoscientific research on the pathological effects of sex hormones on living organisms; and the other concerning the environmental costs of the twentieth century's petrochemical and pharmaceutical industries. The mobilisation of these

---

[3] See, for example, Riley, Bell and Warhurst 1999; Berkson 2000: 81–101; Friends of the Earth 2001a and 2001b.

histories means that even critical environmentalist arguments configure normative sex/gender relations as 'natural' and consequently in need of protection. Rather than using the current moment of crisis in human-animal-environment interimplications to expose the assumptions of 'natural' relationships between these categories, environmentalist, mass media and popular science discourses of endocrine disruptors, as I will show, reproduce heteronormative figurations of both hormones and sex/gender.

Exposure to 'abnormal' levels of hormones: technoscientific histories

Seaman's claim that environmental oestrogens might change 'male humans' into 'women' not only blends sex and gender (referring to 'male humans' and 'women' as if biology and social identity are equally affected by hormones) but also, in her reference to 'an all-female planet', assumes that what keeps everyone from being 'female' is freedom from exposure to oestrogens or other feminising chemicals. These assumptions and concerns have a specific history, one that has been introduced in earlier chapters of this book. Biomedical and technoscientific discourses have long focused on assessing the impact of 'abnormal' levels of hormones on sexed bodies; indeed, like many other sciences, endocrinology has historically produced much of its knowledge about 'normal' (hormonal) systems through studying (hormonally caused) 'pathologies'; early endocrinological work focused on what historian Chandak Sengoopta (1998: 459) calls 'the production of morphological anomalies and other distortions in development'.[4] Throughout the twentieth century, scientists studied the effects of both the deliberate introduction of hormones into human and animal bodies in medicine and experimental science and accidental exposures *in utero* and in later life. In all cases, knowledge produced from 'pathological' examples has been used both to develop understandings of the 'normal' messaging actions of endogenous hormones in producing sex, gender and sexed bodies and to assess the potential and existing dangers of exogenous hormones. As the following brief history shows, this research articulated heteronormative understandings of the relationships between hormones and sex that are carried forward into descriptions of endocrine disruption today.

The 'founding story' of endocrinology – that of Brown-Séquard's self-injection with crushed guinea pig gonads to rejuvenate his sexual drive – initiated a new medical treatment known as organotherapy. Based

---

[4] For examples in other sciences, see Canguilhem 1988; Waldby 1996.

on simple models of sexuality and biological causality, organotherapy advocates asserted that the 'active ingredients' in animal gonads could be transferred to human bodies as a form of replenishment. This late nineteenth-century model was developed in the early twentieth century by Austrian endocrinologist Eugen Steinach who experimented extensively with the transplantation of gonads in rats and guinea pigs. In 1911, this research was extrapolated into the clinical human realm, when Steinach's colleague Robert Lichtenstern (reportedly successfully) transplanted a man's undescended testicle into the abdomen of a solider who had lost his testicles in the war in order to rejuvenate his flagging masculinity (Steinach and Loebel 1940: 96–7). These animal and human experiments supported the new theory that sex was a matter of chemicals rather than nerves. Steinach's experiments also showed that animals undergoing transplantation of gonads of the 'opposite' sex became masculinised in the case of females and feminised in the case of males. His supposition was that male gonads produced a masculinising chemical and female gonads a feminising one. These chemicals, he argued, were also antagonistic to each other. Reporting on his experiments in his later popular account, *Sex and Life*, Steinach wrote, 'the ovary must thus contain, besides the substance which stimulates the development of female attributes, another substance which influences the characteristics of masculinity, but in their opposite direction, causing their repression' (Steinach and Loebel 1940: 92).

In part through his personal association with radical German sexologist Magnus Hirschfeld,[5] Steinach's experiments with animal gonads were closely connected to contemporary sexological attempts to explain 'pathological' sexual behaviours and identities. Hirschfeld believed that endocrinological processes determined sexual orientation and produced homosexuals as a third sex – an intermediate stage between men and women (Wolff 1986: 128–9; Steakley 1997).[6] Providing experimental support for this theory through his

---

[5] Steinach met Hirschfeld in 1914 and became his mentor. According to biographer Janet Wolff, Hirschfeld was 'fascinated by Steinach, whose work complemented his own and was the crowning proof of his theory of sexual intermediaries' (Wolff 1986: 140). The significance of this relationship for the development of endocrinological thought is analysed by Sengoopta (1998 and 2000). Interestingly, Steinach does not discuss this connection in his later account of his life's work (Steinach and Loebel 1940).

[6] The notion of the third sex was originally developed in 1864 by lawyer Karl Ulrichs, who wrote of a third sex called urnings or uranians. Historian Sander Gilman writes, 'Homosexual Jewish scientists such as Magnus Hirschfeld transmuted Ulrich's legal rhetoric into the language of medical science – and the view of the "sexual intermediary classes" was developed. By the 1980s, this view dominated debates within the homosexual emancipation movement' (Gilman 1995: 177).

animal research, Steinach argued that homosexuals were produced by a hermaphroditic or intermediate gland and used this to justify the implanting of the testicular tissue of heterosexual men into homosexual men's bodies. Although these theories and practices suggested that, as Steinach wrote, 'Perfect specimens of a single sex are in reality theoretical ideals; a complete man is as non-existent as a complete woman' (Steinach and Loebel 1940: 113), they did not, Sengoopta (1998) convincingly argues, seriously challenge normative understandings of sexual difference. As a third sex, homosexuals were mixtures of femininity and masculinity, not something outside this dichotomy. As discussed in Chapter 4, at this time the model of health was still one of binary – although no longer biochemically absolute – sexual difference.

Steinach's work was taken up in the United States by embryologist Frank R. Lillie, who, as historical sociologist Adele Clarke argues, 'imported endocrinology into the embryology of his day' by combining the study of hormones with that of genetics (Clarke 1998: 81). This was a unique and important move in the science of sex determination. Studying cattle and particularly sterile females of mixed sex twin pairs (or freemartins), Lillie found in 1916 that exposure to 'male' sex hormones *in utero* caused genetically female embryos to develop male characteristics (Hodann 1937: 19–21). In a 1936 encyclopaedia entry on homosexuality, Hirschfeld summed up his views on Steinach's work, arguing that what was most important about it was the discovery of the role of the gonads in creating sexual difference. 'Steinach's belief ... that he has actually found female cells in the sex glands of homosexual men', he wrote,

> seems to matter less to me than the fact, proved beyond doubt, that male, female and intersexual constitutional types can be created at will by implanting certain sex glands in diverse species of animals. In other words that, like the male and female sex type, the intersexual, in its varied stages, is dependant upon the gonads.
>
> *(Hirschfeld 1936: 334)*

Although this research was eventually discredited through the failure of clinical treatments of homosexuals based upon it, the idea that exogenous (in this case transplanted) gonadal substances could have profound effects on sexual embodiment and behaviours had an enduring impact on endocrinological understandings of sex and sexuality (Sengoopta 1998, 2000; Fausto-Sterling 2000). The emphasis on using animals such as rats and guinea pigs as stand-ins for humans in the study of sex also survived.[7]

---

[7] Steinach claimed to be the first scientist to use rats as experimental animals. He wrote of owing a 'debt of gratitude to the rat' and stated that 'in almost all biological experiment, particularly in hormone research, the rat has since made a place of honour for itself because

After the chemical isolation of hormones in the 1930s, researchers moved from transplanting gonads to injecting hormones or anti-hormones into animals to investigate their physical and behavioural effects. Mid-century research in rodents described a very simple relationship between sex hormones, sex and sexual behaviour: male hormones caused maleness and absence of male hormones caused femaleness. In the 1950s and 1960s, this model was elaborated through the experimental rodent work of Alfred Jost and William C. Young, whose theories are still used today to argue that sex and sexed behaviours are caused by the hormonal activation of a previously established genetic and hormonal physiology (Fausto-Sterling 2000: 195–232). Homosexuality, in this model, 'resulted from prenatal exposure to the wrong quantity or quality of hormone' (Fausto-Sterling 2000: 225).[8] Rodents were not the only animals used to make such arguments – significant bodies of research were also undertaken on birds and primates (Fausto-Sterling 2000: 344, n11).

In her detailed discussion of this research into the behavioural and physiological effects of exogenous sex hormones, Anne Fausto-Sterling (2000: 225) concludes that 'Studies of animal and human sexuality have been hopelessly confused with each other.' This confusion is partly due to ethical restrictions on injecting hormones into humans within purely experimental (non-treatment-related) protocols. The bulk of the literature on hormones and gendered behaviours in humans necessarily focusses on children and adults accidentally exposed to 'abnormal' levels of hormones *in utero*, in particular girls with congenital adrenal hyperplasia and boys with androgen insensitivity disorders. As discussed in Chapter 3, the approach of most of these studies is to measure a particular set of behaviours – anything from children's drawing and musical ability, to play and left-handedness – and to posit a correlation between prenatal hormonal exposure and this behaviour. Many such studies explicitly extend animal studies to humans, relying on early twentieth-century models of homosexuality as a form of behavioural and psychological intersexuality: exposure to testosterone

---

its cooperation, though involuntary, has contributed to countless and important successes' (Steinach and Loebel 1940: 31). Fausto-Sterling (2000: 195–232) provides a fascinating analysis of the historical use of rats and guinea pigs in hormone research, including Steinach's work.

[8] In this chapter of *Sexing the Body*, Fausto-Sterling also describes the work of Frank Beach from the mid-1940s until the 1980s. This research, also undertaken on rodents, pursued a different understanding of sex and sexuality, arguing for an inherent bisexuality underpinning both male and female behaviours. Fausto-Sterling argues that Beach's work represented a less determinist view of rodent (and by implication) human sexuality that was later overshadowed by more heterosexist and conventionally gendered models of Jost and Young.

in utero, for example, is seen to contribute to lesbian sexuality in adult life (McCormick *et al*. 1990; Curtis 2004; Berglund *et al*. 2006). This approach to the study of homosexuality as pathology has demonstrated extraordinary resilience over the twentieth century, becoming a regularly reported (and much criticised) phenomenon in the mass media (Terry 1999).[9] The work of neurologist Simon LeVay (1991, 1993) on so-called 'gay brains', although not based on endocrinological explanations, is exemplary in this respect.[10]

The history of scientific research on the effects of introduced or exogenous hormones on sexed bodies and sexual behaviours is folded into contemporary discourses around environmental oestrogens or endocrine-disrupting chemicals. These discourses animate contemporary debates in several ways: through providing concepts (of the 'naturalness' of binary hormonal sex), practices (of measuring hormones and using animals as models for humans), standards (descriptions of 'normal' and 'pathological' hormonal bodies) and frames through which contemporary data are viewed. Before providing detailed examples of this, however, the next section introduces a second significant historical element of endocrine-disruption discourses.

Environmental histories: toxic chemicals, nature and sex

The second historical antecedent of contemporary discourses on endocrine disruption comes from critical analyses of the toxic effects of the petrochemical and pharmacological industries. Much contemporary writing on endocrine disruption claims roots in Rachel Carson's 1962 classic text, *Silent Spring*. This book is often described as one of the most important books of the twentieth century and is credited with initiating the modern environmental movement (see, for example, McLaughlin 2001). In it,

---

[9] Much critical work in the area of biological accounts of homosexuality is historically based. The work of Foucault (1987), Jeffrey Weeks (1981; 1986) and Jennifer Terry (1999), explores the ways in which connections between sexual practices and sexual identities have been actively made within medical and scientific practices with the complex participation of many homosexual people. As each of these writers makes clear, the understanding of homosexuality as biological, which underpins contemporary endocrinological explanations of sexual preference, developed over the nineteenth and twentieth centuries in tandem with expanding understandings of homosexuality as a form of identity. Despite often being in tension, these two strands assisted each other's progress. As Weeks states, 'The inevitable contradictory effect [of scientific work on homosexuality] was that a growing awareness of homosexuality, an ever-expanding explosion of works about it, accompanied its more detailed organisation and control; and this in turn created the elements of resistance and self-definition that led to the growth of distinctive homosexual identities' (Weeks 1981: 107–8). The mixing of categories of identity and sexual practice in contemporary technoscience is, in part at least, an artefact of this complex history.

[10] For a critique of this work from a biologist, see Rogers 1999: 51–74.

Carson details the extravagances of the mid-twentieth-century agricultural and governmental use of chlorinated hydrocarbons (especially DDT) in the production of food and the control of pests, and the effects of this on plants and animals. In relation to humans, Carson suggests that these chemicals are either directly or indirectly carcinogenic. This indirect route travels, in part at least, via sex hormones. Carson writes:

> A substance that is not a carcinogen in the ordinary sense may disturb the normal functioning of some part of the body in such a way that malignancy results. Important examples are the cancers, especially of the reproductive system, that appear to be linked with disturbances of the balance of sex hormones; these disturbances, in turn, may in some cases be the result of something that affects the ability of the liver to preserve a proper level of these hormones. The chlorinated hydrocarbons are precisely the kind of agent that can bring about this kind of indirect carcinogenesis, because all of them are toxic in some degree to the liver.
>
> *(Carson 1962: 192)*

Chlorinated hydrocarbons, in other words, compromise the liver's ability to maintain normal levels of hormones, which may lead to cancer. Accordingly, Carson cites with approval the description of the western condition as living in a 'sea of carcinogens' (Carson 1962: 196).

It is fascinating to situate Carson's book in endocrinological history. The 1960s was the decade in which Robert A. Wilson began to promote oestrogen-taking for all women over the age of 35 and Wyeth established HRT as a major pharmaceutical product, employing large networks of stables to supply oestrogen-rich equine urine. Concurrently, William C. Young's animal experiments on the endocrinological aspects of sex were interpreted to indicate the viability of a continuum model of human gender differences in which 'pathologies' such as intersexuality could, as in the clinical work of John Money and Anke Ehrhardt, be 'treated'. It was also, importantly, the decade in which the first surgeries (and related hormonal treatments) for transsexuality were attempted (Irvine 1990: 258–66). In contrast to all this optimism about biomedical hormonal intervention, then, *Silent Spring* articulates prescient concern about exogenous chemicals and the environmental and health-related costs of technoscientific 'progress'. Today, this concern is attached to endocrine disruptors.

Contemporary discourses of endocrine disruption: mobilising hormone histories

These two material-semiotic histories are mobilised in contemporary discourses of endocrine disruption. Billed in its preface as the successor to

Silent Spring and commonly cited as the most important popular book on endocrine-disrupting chemicals, Theo Colborn, Dianne Dumanoski and John Peterson Myers' 1996 book, *Our Stolen Future: are we threatening our fertility, intelligence, and survival?*, provides an excellent initial example.[11] In a chapter pointedly entitled 'Beyond cancer', Colborn and colleagues criticise the 'scientific establishment's' focus since *Silent Spring* on the role of chemicals in producing cancer (Colborn *et al.* 1996: 198–209). Endocrine-disrupting chemicals, they argue, do not act in the same way as carcinogens and are not poisons in the normal sense: 'Until we recognise this', they assert, 'we will be looking in the wrong places [and] asking the wrong questions' (Colborn *et al.* 1996: 203). In line with much contemporary biomedical thinking, *Our Stolen Future* describes the hormonal body as informational; figuring endocrine-disrupting chemicals as 'the thugs on the biological information highway that sabotage vital communication' (Colborn *et al.* 1996: 203).[12] Playing on the scientific metaphor of hormones as messengers, endocrine-disrupting chemicals are said to 'mug the messengers, or impersonate them. They jam signals. They scramble messages. They sow information' (Colborn *et al.* 1996: 203). In direct contradiction of Carson, Colborn and colleagues stress that today, 'The key concept in thinking about this kind of toxic assault is ... [n]ot poisons, not carcinogens, but chemical messages' (Colborn *et al.* 1996: 204). This focus on the message-disrupting abilities of these chemicals shifts attention away from cancer towards sexual reproduction. Colborn *et al.* argue that, 'What is at stake [now] is not simply a matter of some individual destinies or impacts on the most sensitive amongst us but a widespread erosion of human potential over the past half century' (Colborn *et al.* 1996: 232).

Colborn and colleagues' argument is emotive, panic-inducing and powerful. These effects are in part dependent on the mobilisation of historical and culturally pervasive understandings of sexual differences as antagonistic, and of human and other animal existence as based on sexual reproduction. The mobilisation of these understandings is evident when Colborn and colleagues evoke the 'insidious erosion of the human species'

---

[11] *Our Stolen Future* also has a wide-ranging website that keeps the interested public up-to-date with the latest research in this field (see www.ourstolenfuture.org. Last accessed 25 September 2006). This website also provides the authors with a space in which they can refute criticisms of their text.

[12] Several cultural analysts of technoscience and biomedicine describe the ways in which bodies came to be understood in terms of information and communication technologies in the second part of the twentieth century. See, for example, Martin 1995 and Haraway 1991: 203–30 in relation to the immune system; Keller 2001 and Kay 2000 in relation to genetics; and Stacey 1997 and 2000 in relation to cancer and alternative health discourses.

potentiated by endocrine-disrupting chemicals (Colborn *et al.* 1996: 234). In an insidious move of their own, Colborn and colleagues suggest that the current 'breakdown of the family', including rising rates of child abuse and neglect and the high rates of attention deficit hyperactivity disorder amongst children, may be caused by endocrine-disrupting chemicals (Colborn *et al.* 1996: 186, 237). Indeed, the action of endocrine-disrupting chemicals is discussed as an 'assault on our children' (Colborn at al 1996: 238).[13] Colborn and colleagues thus amplify the threat of endocrine disruption with reference to psychobiology, behavioural psychology and psychoneuroendocrinology (specifically LeVay's work on the biological causes of homosexuality) and by neglecting the role of social forces in human sexuality, family relationships and child abuse and children's behaviour. Reliance on such research means that ultimately, despite paying lip service to the importance of social factors in the production of human sexuality (Colborn *et al.* 1996: 194–5), Colborn and colleagues state: '[W]e are confident that ongoing research will confirm that the hormonal experience of the developing embryo at crucial stages of its development has an impact on adult behaviour in humans, affecting the choice of mates, parenting, social behaviour, and other significant dimensions of humanity' (Colborn *et al.* 1996: 238). Such confidence is based on a long history of speculation, founded on problematic technoscientific knowledges.

Another book hailed on its back cover as the successor to *Silent Spring* is D. Lindsey Berkson's (2000) *Hormone Deception*. As a consulting scholar at environmental toxicologist John McLachlan's research centre, Berkson has a strong connection to technoscientific work in this field, although she is not a scientist herself. Her book repackages contemporary technoscientific research for the worried consumer, combining this with a range of alternative health discourses. Like Colborn and colleagues, Berkson uses the technoscientific metaphor of messaging, citing a scientist speaking at a 1997 UN conference on environment and development in the epigraph to her first chapter:

> When you think about it, life is about messages. What I am referring to here are the natural chemical messages that come from our genes and become the instructions for the next generation: how to grow, how to develop, how to mature from fetus to adulthood. These messages are life itself.
>
> *(Myers, quoted in Berkson 2000: 3)*

---

[13] Greenpeace also use the word 'assault' to describe the effects of endocrine disruptors on children (Dorey 2003: 8).

Hormones, Berkson consequently suggests, are 'messengers of life' (the title of her chapter).

Again, like Colborn and colleagues, Berkson uses the messenger metaphor and its associations with secrecy and potential sabotage to provoke concern in her readers. Describing the actions of endocrine disruptors, she writes, 'Hormone disruptors that gain entry into the human body can act like saboteurs who enter a top-secret government installation and download a virus into the communications software' (Berkson 2000: 48). Endocrine disruptors are figured here as destructive hackers, working to undermine the state – in the current socio-political context where fear of viral contamination of information and communication technologies is high, this is an affective analogy.

The insidious, destructive labour of endocrine disruptors becomes even more disturbing and particularly poignant when Berkson describes her own experience as a 'DES daughter'. Diethylstilbestrol (DES) is a synthetic oestrogen that was prescribed to millions of pregnant women from 1938 to 1971 to prevent miscarriage and support a healthy pregnancy.[14] Prescribed before any controlled studies had been undertaken, DES had severe consequences for the children of the women who took it. Many daughters (and some sons) of these women developed reproductive tract cancers and other serious health problems after puberty. Berkson (2000: 61) describes a terrible list of personal health problems attributed to her mother's DES-taking, including breast cancer, infertility and severely painful endometriosis leading to ovarectomy.

In the form of DES, exogenous sex hormones are patently extremely toxic chemicals. Their effects are also transgenerational: not only the daughters and sons, but now also the grandchildren of women who took DES during pregnancy are understood to be at increased risk of cancer and other illnesses (Newbold *et al* 1998).[15] DES was also extensively fed to animals raised for meat until the 1970s and was thus consumed by millions of humans and domesticated carnivores. Much American meat, according to Berkson (2000: 67), still contains similar compounds, known as oestrogenic growth promoters. All of this consumption of oestrogenic substances, Berkson argues, challenges human reproductivity, producing infertility in serious cases like her own. Discussion of this leads Berkson on to

---

[14] Five million women took DES in the United States alone (Berkson 2000: 61).

[15] Recent research on the effects of toxic chemicals (in this case a fungicide used in the wine industry) in mice also indicate that effects on reproductive systems can perpetuate across several generations (Anway *et al* 2005).

more speculative territory, linking her writing to histories of endocrinological research into human sexuality. 'This leads to an interesting question', she writes,

> could exposure to endocrine disruptors lead to homosexuality? Many sex-
> related characteristics are determined by hormones during the early stages of
> development, and they can be influenced by very small changes in hormonal
> balance. A controlled DES study run by a university showed a statistically
> significant (beyond chance) correlation between being a DES daughter and
> lesbianism. Evidence suggests that once sex-related characteristics are
> imprinted, they may be irreversible.
>
> *(Berkson 2000: 135)*

As in Colborn and colleagues' case, such speculation confirms a heteronormative orientation in which heterosexuality is 'caused' by hormonal action.
This normativity is confirmed by the title of the immediately following
section of *Hormone Deception*: 'There are never enough good men.'[16]

The emphasis on endocrine-disrupting chemicals as a threat to human
sexual reproduction is not limited to popular books. Well-known environmental groups, such as the WWF, Friends of the Earth and Greenpeace,
have produced policy statements, reports and awareness-raising campaigns on endocrine-disrupting chemicals.[17] Whilst containing much valuable technoscientific information and political argumentation, these
documents also mobilise cultural norms in order to provoke concern and
action around endocrine disruptors. In numerous places, as I will show,
this mobilisation becomes quite troubling: the documents rely on problematic representations of women's bodies, foetuses and sexed responsibilities
for caring for children's and others' health.

The World Wildlife Fund for Nature (WWF) has a strong connection to
Colborn, who wrote *Our Stolen Future* in her capacity as 'WWF's senior
scientist' (WWF 1998). Many WWF publications, then, contain a similar
rhetoric to that of *Our Stolen Future*. In their report, 'Chemicals that
compromise life: a call to action', for example, WWF write that 'Whatever
the mechanism, the bottom line is always the same: Any chemical that

---

[16] The section is about sex ratios at birth, but Berkson jokes that 'many of us think there
aren't enough men as it is' (Berkson 2000: 136).

[17] See for WWF: 1998; 1999; 2006; for Friends of the Earth: Riley, Bell and Warhurst 1999;
Warhurst 2000; Friends of the Earth 2001d; and for Greenpeace: Greenpeace 2003; 2005;
Thornton 1997. In 2005, these campaigns focused on an important vote in the European
Union around the regulation of chemicals, known as REACH (Registration, Evaluation
and Authorisation of Chemicals). Despite intense campaigning, environmental groups
were disappointed by the final outcome, which leaves many potentially dangerous chemicals unregulated.

interferes with hormones can scramble vital messages, derail development, and undermine health' (WWF 1998: 2). This use of emotive language is amplified in the WWF's awareness-raising campaigns on endocrine-disrupting chemicals. One example published in UK newspapers, magazines and on the internet in February 2002, aims to provoke a strong response (see Figure 1). Utilising a red-tinted close-up of a human foetus, the full-page advertisement states, 'The womb should be the safest place on earth. But today our bodies are contaminated with over 300 man-made chemicals, to which our great-grandparents were never exposed ... The WWF is campaigning for the elimination of these hazardous chemicals, so that the only thing we pass on to our children is our genes' (WWF 2002). From a feminist perspective, the use of this image is highly problematic. Invoking both anti-abortion politics (in which the use of similar images to evoke the vulnerability of the foetus is commonplace) and a restrictive figuration of mothers as 'place' or environment, this image unavoidably – even if unintentionally – ties WWF's work on endocrine-disrupting chemicals with right-wing, anti-feminist campaigns around issues of reproduction.[18]

Other environmental NGOs also employ images of pregnant women and foetuses to illustrate the dangers of endocrine disruptors. Greenpeace's 2005 web-based report, *Poisoning the Unborn*, for example, uses an illustration of a naked pregnant woman lying along the bottom of a spherical window, gazing away into a blue, oceanic scene of (presumably) toxic water. 'Our children inherit the toxic burden of our planet', the accompanying text declares. Figured as a foetus lying in the womb of the world (living, it seems, 'in a sea of oestrogens'), this woman – like the foetus of the WWF advertisement – represents vulnerability and purity, but is also a conduit, passing on toxicity through her bloodstream to her 'unborn child'. This figuration of women as 'natural' conduits reproduces conventional understandings of sex/gender in which women's central importance is as mothers rather than subjects in their own right.

Environmental NGOs also cite problematic histories of endocrinological research. In a longer report entitled 'Human impacts of man-made chemicals' (which uses an image of a cropped pregnant woman's body on the title page), Greenpeace lists as one of the 'range of health problems' associated with 'commonly used chemicals', 'the feminisation of young boys and the masculinisation of girls' (Greenpeace 2003: 2). Citing Dutch

---

[18] For feminist work on the image of the foetus and its connections to anti-abortion politics and the representation of mothers as environments, see Duden 1993; Haraway 1997; Hartouni 1997.

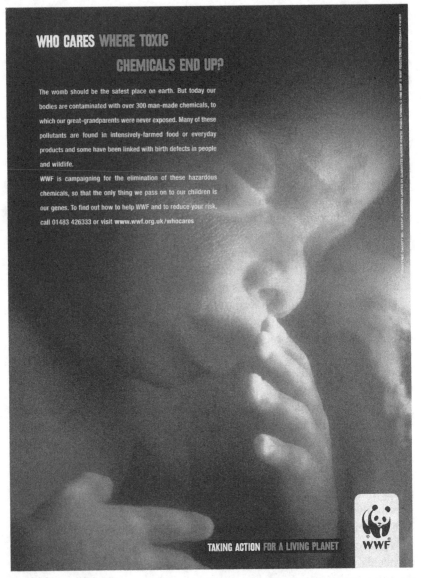

Figure 1. WWF 'Who cares where toxic chemicals end up?' Campaign advertisement

research on children's schoolyard behaviour (Vreughenhil *et al.* 2002), the report suggests that 'exposure to PCBs and dioxins significantly affect the types of play youngsters engage in ... Boys exposed to PCBs in the womb tend to engage in more feminine play. Girls exposed to PCBs become more masculine. Dioxin exposure leads to both girls and boys becoming more feminine' (Greenpeace 2003: 8). Stemming historically from the animal experiments of the early twentieth century, such research is based on highly problematic assumptions about the relationship between sexed biologies and gendered behaviours and involves heteronormative assumptions about what sort of behaviours are 'typical' for boys and not for girls and vice versa, suggesting both that girls and boys are naturally 'opposites' and that what is 'typical' is therefore biologically based.[19] In the original Dutch study, for example, Vreugdenhil *et al.* discuss the results of another study of children whose mothers were exposed to extreme levels of PCBs and PCDFs (dioxins) that found exposed boys had poor spatial abilities: 'Because boys typically develop better spatial abilities than girls', they write, 'these results were interpreted as demasculinizing or feminising effects caused by disturbances in steroid hormones by prenatal exposure to PCBs/PCDFs' (Vreugdenhil *et al* 2002: 596). This quote epitomises both problems: it assumes that boys showing fewer masculine behaviours are feminised *and* that this decline must be caused by biological factors (there could, of course, be many social explanations of boys' decrease in spatial abilities). In this simplistic approach to gender and behaviour, this tech-noscientific work is reminiscent of the popular books of Steve Biddulph and Simon Baron-Cohen discussed in earlier chapters. Both discourses naturalise conventional modes of gendered embodiment and behaviour, naming difference (or lack of it, in terms of binary sexual difference) as pathological.

In recent years, key governmental and scientific bodies in the USA (National Research Council 1999), Britain (The Royal Society 2000) and other countries have produced documents summarising current research and making strong calls for more work in this area (see Krimsky 2000). This scientific literature is, unsurprisingly, less dramatic in its claims about the impact of endocrine-disrupting chemicals on human reproductive capacities, arguing, for example, that declines in sperm count have yet to be finally demonstrated (National Research Council 1999: 4) and that the biological routes of endocrine-disrupting chemicals' actions remain under-explicated. The Royal Society document speaks of 'speculation' in this field and states that 'many questions about EDCs [endocrine-disrupting

---

[19] Vreugdenhil *et al.*'s study claims to be the first behavioural study of the effects of endocrine disruptors in humans. The study has other methodological problems including the fact that play behaviour is assessed by the children's parents (their mothers in 84 per cent of cases) (Vreugdenhil *et al* 2002: 595). Most parents are arguably highly motivated to see their children's behaviour as gender-normal and are thus more likely to 'see' and report the behaviours they find acceptable.

chemicals] cannot be answered yet' (The Royal Society 2000: 1–2). Despite this cautious tone, the experience of DES daughters remains a strong spectre in this literature, provoking concern that the role of endocrine disruptors be further monitored and studied: 'Continued research is essential if the uncertainties are to be properly addressed and the risks understood', The Royal Society (2000: 2) document states.

The gap between the more sober rhetoric of governmental and scientific bodies and the emotive appeals of the NGO literature is predictable – these are, after all, quite different genres, articulating significantly different interests. These differences are, however, exacerbated by the nature of the technoscientific field itself, which is, as toxicologist John McLachlan writes, 'rife with debate, inconsistencies, and controversy' (McLachlan 2001: 320; see also Krimsky 2000). In part this can be ascribed to the multidisciplinary nature of the field, but McLachlan also stresses the importance of intense public and regulatory debates to this area, stating that 'The regulatory and media interest in the topic often move at a faster pace than the science' (McLachlan 2001: 320). Unusually in a scientific literature review, McLachlan refers to both the publication of *Our Stolen Future* and the Emmy award winning documentary, *Assault on the Male* by Deborah Cadbury (author of *The Feminization of Nature: our future at risk*, a very similar book to Colborn *et al.* and Berkson) and claims that the public interest voiced in these texts has 'driven, or at least influenced' scientific work in this field (McLachlan 2001: 320).

Whilst this claim of media and regulatory interest running ahead of the science problematically makes a distinction between 'the science' and its popular and regulatory lives,[20] McLachlan is right to point out the significant role of the media in producing interest in endocrine disruption. As was argued in Chapter 3 in relation to research on hormones and behaviour, science and medical journalism does provide a bridge between technoscientific research and popular discourses, articulating a set of frames through which technoscientific research is rendered accessible to the public. In the case of endocrine disruptors, these frames have their roots in the two material-semiotic histories described earlier; roots that are evident in their mobilisation of panic-inducing claims about the effects of endocrine disruptors on sex and reproduction. In a two-part series published in *Science News*, for example, Janet Raloff (1994a, 1994b) writes that

---

[20] Interestingly, in many fields of contemporary technoscience the opposite claim is made: that the science is running ahead of public opinion and regulation. For a critical discussion of this in relation to the genetic testing of embryos see Franklin and Roberts 2006.

'Mother Nature is exerting a feminising hormonal influence' on both human and non-human animals, suggesting, like Barbara Seaman, that 'With the growing ubiquity of pesticides and other pollutants possessing the functional attributes of female hormones, our environment effectively bathes us in a sea of oestrogens' (Raloff 1994b: 56). A series of full-colour supplements entitled *Chemical World* published in the *Guardian* in 2004 also articulates a sense of doom, using extreme close-up images of everyday food and household items to suggest that familiar items harbour unfamiliar and dangerous chemicals and that foods that regulators say are safe may not be because 'no testing of the effects of pesticides in combination is required or performed' (Moorhead 2004: 21). Although these articles are also full of advice about how to minimise exposure to endocrine-disrupting chemicals, their overall effect is to produce a sense of widespread, unavoidable contamination. Like the NGO campaigns, these articles also use images of foetuses to illustrate the dangers of endocrine disruption. A *Guardian* article entitled 'Food Chained', for example, is framed by an extreme close-up of a foetus and umbilical cord. Unlike the other pictures in the article, this image is uncaptioned – it apparently speaks for itself – but the text cites foetal toxicologist Vyvyan Howard claiming that 'We have changed the chemical environment of the womb', and arguing that these changes are linked to increased cancer rates in children and adults (Lawrence 2004: 7).

The fundamental assertion of these popular and mass media discourses on the effects of endocrine disruptors is that 'we' may no longer be 'us'. Using powerful images of vulnerable foetuses and alarmist language, they suggest that the effects of environmental oestrogens on male reproductive systems spell the end of sexual reproduction and sex and thus humanity itself (recall Berkson's epigraph that referred to hormones as 'life itself'). UK science journalist Deborah Cadbury, author of *The Feminization of Nature*, for example, writes that 'Some scientists argue that ... *it will not be long before human reproduction will be under threat*' (Cadbury 1998: x, emphasis added). Likewise, Colborn and colleagues gravely state that 'the danger we face is not simply death and disease. By disrupting hormones and development, these synthetic chemicals *may be changing who we become*' (1996: 197, emphasis added). The WWF similarly warns that 'The mounting scientific evidence confronts us with disturbing questions about the extent to which hormonally active chemicals are altering our children's ability to learn, to function in a social environment, to resist disease, and to reproduce. *The integrity of the next generation is on the line.* Our response should reflect the true magnitude of these stakes' (1998: 8, emphasis added), whilst Berkson claims that 'hormone disruption can possibly affect everything from lowered sperm count to our ability to fight off diseases. *It can alter or determine our and our children's destiny*' (2000: xxiii, emphasis added). These claims are heteronormative: relying on long histories of problematic technoscientific research into the effects of hormones on sexed bodies and behaviours, they articulate heterosexuality and binary sexual difference as healthy norms. Like many forms of nostalgia, they refer to a past that never existed; in this case, one constituted by intact biological and social boundaries between male and female human and non-human animals, flawless reproductivity and a clear sense of biologically based, sexed human identities.

Feminism and the politics of endocrine disruption

Developing a feminist response to discourses on endocrine-disrupting chemicals is challenging, in part because these discourses bring us sharply up against a set of technoscientific claims about the possible effects of exogenous hormones on bodies. Feminist biologist Lynda Birke (one of the only feminists writing on this topic) describes herself as 'fence-sitting' when analysing environmental oestrogens (Birke 2000). On one side of the fence, she is critical of discourse around 'gender-bending chemicals', arguing that they make a number of problematic assumptions about gender and nature. On the other side, she feels compelled to adopt a 'realist' position in relation to the scientific evidence presented about the material effects of endocrine disruptors on bodies. Ultimately she calls her fence-sitting position 'contingent realism', arguing that it is possible both to draw on scientific data as a resource *and* 'play the social constructionist game and unpick the categories by which we understand, say, gender' (Birke 2000: 596).

I am more optimistic than Birke about the resources feminist theory and science studies have to offer to a critical analysis of endocrine-disrupting chemicals. Combining the substantial feminist literature on sex, sexuality and gender with a critical approach to biology, allows an understanding of endocrine-disrupting chemicals that can acknowledge the material effects of such chemicals and also remain critical of the ways in which these actions are figured in different discourses. Extending the notion of hormones as messengers of sex to include chemicals that act like hormones (endocrine disruptors) provides a route into such an analysis. Using this idea makes possible an analysis that resonates with Judith Butler's important aphorism about sex: 'There may not be a materiality of sex that is not already burdened by the sex of materiality' (Butler 1993: 54). Descriptions of 'sex', like those made by popular writers, environmentalists or scientists, always fold in previous histories of this concept (Butler suggests that materiality itself is understood as feminine). This folding – or burdening, to use Butler's term – is both material and semiotic; it is bio-social. Histories of research into endocrinological sex are evident in descriptions of hormonally disrupted bodies (alligators with small penises, seagulls nesting in 'lesbian' pairs) and in questions asked about endocrine-disrupting chemicals (Do they cause homosexuality? Might they morph men into women?). Material histories of sex are also literally embodied in relation to endocrine disruptors: women like Berkson, whose mothers took DES, suffer the physical consequences of these actions, as do those who eat the meat of cattle or pigs fed with oestrogenic growth promoters. Consuming endocrine-disrupting chemicals in meat, we ingest historically specific, materialised hormone-related theories and ideas (oestrogen causes beneficial, non-toxic growth in animals) and practices (injections of hormonal extracts), and materially encounter the consequences of these histories in and as our bodies. In thinking about endocrine disruption, in other words, it is evident that sex is both semiotic and material and always historically situated.

The materiality of sex today is in part enacted through the action of endocrine disruptors. But this materiality is always 'burdened' by the material-semiotic histories of endocrinology: its production of sex through material-semiotic practices of transplanting gonads, injecting animals and scientifically studying human bodies and behaviours. There is no need, in this analysis, to fence-sit in the way Birke describes; indeed there is no fence, because there can never be a divide between 'the real' material effects of endocrine disruptors and the problematic discourses that describe them. In Chapter 5, I argued along similar lines that it is not possible to disentangle the biological effects of HRT on menopausal women's bodies from medical and other discourses about women's 'pathological' differences from men, the idea of aging as a pathology and cultural ideas about sex and sexuality. The 'real' effects of HRT, like the 'real' effects of endocrine disruptors, are always intertwined or entangled with other material-semiotic factors: these effects are the results of such entanglements, not isolated or independent facts. Such entanglement is intrinsic to my refiguring of the phrase 'messengers of sex'. As messengers, hormones do not carry an independent entity from one place to another, but create a kind of relationality in which their messaging activities constitute the entities that they are thought to message between. This relationality is suggested by the hyphen in bio-social, which represents a constituting, active relation between two entities (the biological and the social) that do not pre-exist on their own but are constituted through their connection with each other (in this case, a connection made through hormones).

Global messaging

Prevalent discourses of endocrine disruption message heteronormative ideas about sex. Mobilising problematic histories of endocrine research, they figure hormones as key actors in producing reproductive heterosexual bodies, families and sexual practices. In some technoscientific narratives, however, we get a glimpse of a more disruptive view of hormones as messengers. In his review of the scientific literature on endocrine-disrupting chemicals, for example, McLachlan uses the concept of hormones as messengers to explain the problems these chemicals pose in the early twenty-first century. 'Environmental signals are chemical messenger molecules', he writes, 'functioning in a communication network linking numerous species ... Chemicals that alter ... levels of information flow can have consequences that may be deleterious to the individual or population' (McLachlan 2001: 335). 'From an environmental stewardship perspective', he continues,

> the evolving concept of environmental signals can provide insights with which to address the impact of hormonally active chemicals on humans and the ecosystems that they share with other species. Disruption of this apparently broad communication system has the potential for global change that transcends the endocrine system.
>
> *(McLachlan 2001: 336)*

McLachlan here uses the messenger concept to press home the global environmental issue at stake: that endocrine-disrupting chemicals effect much more than human endocrine systems. Pushed to its limits, this point reconfigures understandings of hormones as messengers; sex hormones are no longer contained in homeostatic biological systems, but 'transcend' these, describing the extent of the 'ecosystems that ... [humans] share with other species'.

The significance of this reconfiguration is evident in technoscientific representations of hormonal messaging systems. In Chapter 2, I discussed textbook representations of the ways in which hormones message sex in human bodies. These representations usually consist of simple line drawings of sexed bodies or diagrammatic flowcharts depicting hormonal pathways as arrows linking neurological and reproductive systems. The endocrine glands in these images are discrete entities, contained within

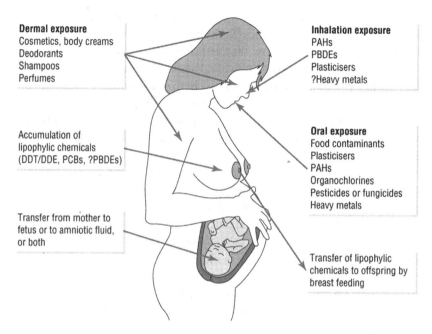

Dermal exposure
Cosmetics, body creams
Deodorants
Shampoos
Perfumes

Inhalation exposure
PAHs
PBDEs
Plasticisers
?Heavy metals

Accumulation of
lipophylic chemicals
(DDT/DDE, PCBs, ?PBDEs)

Oral exposure
Food contaminants
Plasticisers
PAHs
Organochlorines
Pesticides or fungicides
Heavy metals

Transfer from mother to
fetus or to amniotic fluid,
or both

Transfer of lipophylic
chemicals to offspring by
breast feeding

Figure 2. The assaulted endocrine body
Source: Richard M. Sharpe and D. Stewart Irvine 'How strong is the evidence of a link
between environmental chemicals and adverse effects on human reproductive health?'
British Medical Journal (328) (21 February 2004): 447–51. Reproduced with permission
from the BMJ Publishing Group Ltd

the boundary of adult humans' skin or the closed systems of the flowcharts'
boxes. In their review article on endocrine-disrupting chemicals, Sharpe
and Irvine produce a new version of this diagram (see Figure 2). Here, the
line drawing of the female body does not consist of a series of internal
pathways maintaining hormonal homeostasis, but is a body subjected to
numerous *external* endocrine exposures. Hormones – again represented by
arrows – enter the body from the outside and are transferred from the
woman (who is, of course, pregnant) to her foetus.[21] This disrupting image
is also represented in popular books. In *Hormone Deception*, for example,
Berkson (2002: 12, 33, 214) uses illustrations of internal 'natural' hormonal
activity (human figures containing arrows) and an image of 'unnatural
environmental signalling ... coming from synthetic sources outside our

---

[21] Resonating with the use of foetal images to depict the dangers of environmental oestrogens
discussed above, this image figures women as conduits of hormonal dangers, placing them
in positions of responsibility towards the hormonal bodies of their (potential) children.

bodies' that depicts a pregnant woman and small child being assaulted by arrows from outside their bodies (Berkson 2002: 33).

These representations show that as messengers of sex, endocrine disruptors transgress the limits of individual bodies. Hormones and chemicals that act like hormones now move across bodies, disrupting boundaries of geography, species and time: they are, as the WWF puts it, 'global travellers' (WWF 1999: 6). The unsettling nature of such moves is represented in a recent public education campaign produced by the British WWF in collaboration with the Cooperative Bank (a British bank that invests ethically). This campaign was published in the *Guardian*'s glossy weekend supplement on the same date as one of their *Chemical World* supplements mentioned above. The campaign depicts a heterosexual family in an English suburban kitchen, eating a conventional breakfast of boiled eggs, toast, cereal and tea. The mother and daughter are dressed in pink and white. The father and son are in blue. The mother is not sitting down, but joins the family only to 'pose' for the picture, implying that she is serving the meal, rather than eating it. The only thing that is non-normative about this family is that they have polar bear heads (polar bears are, of course, white) (see Figure 3). The text asks: 'Polar bears don't live in houses, so why have chemicals from houses been found in their bodies? Polar bears live in the Arctic, about as far away from your average semi-detached as you can get. So why do chemicals more commonly found in carpets, curtains, cleaning products and even games consoles contaminate their bodies?' (Cooperative Bank and WWF 2004).

This campaign refers to scientific findings that endocrine-disrupting chemicals originating in the southern hemisphere have been found in the fat of polar bears in the Arctic Circle. This fat is consumed by Inuit children in Canada and Alaska, who are subsequently at risk of developmental and reproductive problems, as are the polar bears themselves. Not only is the Inuit's food source under threat because of the reproductive impact of endocrine-disrupting chemicals on polar bears, but their own children's health and reproductive futures may also share a similar fate if they continue to consume this staple food.[22] The Cooperative Bank and WWF campaign, however, does not refer to these issues of polar bear reproductivity, Inuit food sources, or the effects on Inuit people of eating this fat. Instead, it uses polar bears to emphasise that '[if endocrine-disrupting chemicals are] turning up in polar bears thousands of miles away, it's no surprise that humans are being contaminated as well'

[22] See Krimsky 2000: 229–30; Solomon and Schletter 2000: 1473; de Bendern 2002.

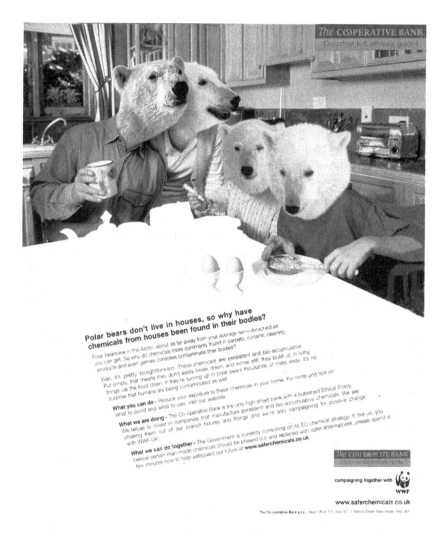

Figure 3. Co-operative Bank and WWF polar-bear–human hybrids. Campaign advertisement

(Cooperative Bank and WWF 2004). 'Humans' in this instance are represented by a normative or 'average' English family, who are unknowingly linked to (or even becoming) polar bears.

This campaign illustrates both the transgressive potential of endocrine disruptors and the ways in which figurations of their global messaging actions reductively undermine this potential. Importantly, the campaign provides an image for the new hormonal body, in which boundaries

pertaining to species, time, geography and bodies are breached by exogenous hormones' messaging actions. The hybrid polar-bear–humans represent this new form of boundary crossing and the accompanying text tells us
that endocrine-disrupting chemicals are flowing literally from one end of
the earth to the other, 'turning up in polar bears thousands of miles away'.
Rather than utilising the transgressive potential of this representation,
however, this campaign mobilises conventional models of kinship and
sexuality in trying to address the potentially serious implications of these
chemicals on human and animal health.

These polar-bear–human hybrids present a significant challenge to
critical thinking about hormonal action; despite its normative align-
ments, the campaign raises serious questions about the global politics
of endocrine disruptors. As cyborgian creatures – literal mixtures of
humans and animals – the polar-bear–human hybrids evoke the work
of Donna Haraway, specifically her analysis of another millennial
cyborg, OncoMouse™. OncoMouse™ is a laboratory animal genetically engineered to reliably develop breast cancer and used as a tool
to research cancer and its treatments in humans. Patented in 1988,
OncoMouse™ is technically an invention and is owned by DuPont, a
world-leading industrial chemical company. This mouse – referred to by
Haraway (1997: 83) as a 'little murine smart bomb' and a 'tool-weapon' –
materially embodies contemporary connections between genomics, cancer and endocrine disruption: s/he is genetically engineered to develop
breast cancer; is owned by a company that has long been involved in the
production of endocrine-disrupting substances; and is a tool in the
investigation of toxic chemicals and their role in producing cancer of
the mammary glands (not only was OncoMouse™ engineered as a biological model for breast cancer, as described by Haraway, s/he was also
'engineered to exhibit heightened sensitivity to toxic substances, allowing
researchers to study carcinogenic environmental factors' (Shorett 2002)).
OncoMouse™, in Haraway's terms, is both a tool and a trope; a being
that reconfigures biological knowledge, laboratory practice, property law
and collective and personal hopes and fears around cancer (Haraway
1997: 79–85). S/he symbolises both the frightening, corporate production
of non-normative bodies *and* the promise of recovery from toxicity-
induced pathology.

Most significant for theorising the polar-bear–human hybrids is
Haraway's argument about the suffering of OncoMouse™. As a stand-
in for humans in laboratory experiments, she suggests, OncoMouse™ –
like Christ in the Christian story of redemption – is sacrificed so that 'we'

can live longer and better. Such sacrifices occur in vast numbers: according to the University of California Davis Cancer Centre (2003), 40 million transgenic mice are used worldwide in cancer research each year. Scientists use genetically engineered mice like OncoMouse[TM] because they are like us (they can represent or stand in for humans), but also because they are not like us (otherwise we would not tolerate this use). This fact, Haraway (1997: 82) argues, means that we are responsible for representing genetically engineered mice in ways that acknowledge their unique status as laboratory animals, surrogates and scapegoats and recognise their significant difference from other scientific tools used in the laboratory. This mode of ethically responsible representation is linked to a mode of articulation with these animals that refuses to reproduce a language of purity or nature, acknowledging that the OncoMouse[TM] is both nature and not nature: an animal whose 'natural habitat' is the laboratory. 'It will not help – emotionally, intellectually, morally, or politically', Haraway argues, 'to appeal to the natural and the pure' in thinking about cyborg entities like the OncoMouse[TM] (Haraway 1997: 62).

In developing these new articulations, Haraway insists that 'We must cast our lot with some ways of life on this planet, and not with other ways' (Haraway 1997: 51). She calls for an ethopolitics that asks questions about the significance and meaning of animal, human and other suffering and makes assessments of the kind of practices or articulations that create the worlds we inhabit (see also Braidotti 2006). 'Following Susan Leigh Star's (1991) lead', Haraway writes,

> the question I want to ask my sibling species, a breast-endowed cyborg like me, is simple: *Cui bono?* For whom does OncoMouse[TM] live and die? If s/he is a figure in the strong sense, then s/he collects up the whole people. S/he is significant. That makes such a question as *cui bono?* unavoidable. Who lives and dies – human, nonhuman, and cyborg – and how, because OncoMouse[TM] exists?
>
> *(Haraway 1997: 113)*[23]

This attitude emphasises relationality without sentimentality and is not one linked in any simple way with an animal rights perspective. Describing the OncoMouse[TM] as like herself, Haraway, it seems, would support the use of OncoMouse[TM] in cancer research as long this use

---

[23] Science-studies theorist Susan Leigh Star (1991) writes about being allergic to onions and the difficulties this causes her when eating at McDonalds' outlets. Haraway borrows the Latin phrase 'Cui bono?' meaning 'Good for whom?' from this article. This phrase denotes a standard rule used in criminal investigations to emphasise that investigators should search for perpetrators amongst those who might benefit from a crime.

'contribute[s] to deeper equality, keener appreciation of heterogeneous multiplicity, and stronger accountability for liveable worlds' (Haraway 1997: 113). (The question of whether current use does this is left unanswered in her book.)

Haraway's analysis of OncoMouse^{TM} provides a frame for thinking about the polar-bear–human hybrids and endocrine-disrupting chemicals. Rather than posing questions about endocrine disruption in terms of purity or natural sexual differences, critics could ask about the kinds of lives 'we' (humans and non-humans) want to have and to reproduce. Changing the questions about endocrine disruptors in this way would mean addressing hormonal bodies in terms that engage critically with the histories of sex that are mobilised around and through them. In its most simple terms, this means developing forms of engagement with the problem of endocrine disruption – such as the problem of breast cancer described by Haraway – that neither rejects nor sacralises technoscience.

In analysing the OncoMouse^{TM} and other contemporary actors such as 'the foetus' and 'the gene', Haraway (1997: 112) selects the terms 'engagement' or 'commitment' rather than 'choice' to describe a preferred relation to contemporary technoscience. She wants to engage with a technoscience that is not about pure nature or culture but is rather an arena in which the implosion of these categories is accepted, an arena of material-semiotic and situated (grounded or worldly) practices: 'Commitment after the implosions of technoscience', she writes, 'requires immersion in the work of materializing new tropes in an always contingent practice of grounding or worlding' (Haraway 1997: 113). Now is the time to engage with biology, she argues, as its importance to all aspects of life continues to grow. I am perhaps less optimistic than Haraway about the chances we have for making significant interventions into this world, but remain nonetheless convinced that feminist politics today has to take place at the level of everyday practices of engaging with technoscience: from taking personal decisions about what to eat and to wear, through reading, thinking and writing about technoscience and biomedicine, to becoming active in relation to working in, through or in relation to technoscience and biomedicine. Answers to the 'Who lives and dies?' questions in the field of endocrine disruption will only come from paying serious critical attention to the ways in which the biological continues to matter to sex, sexuality and sexual reproduction. This attention also opens up more traditionally political questions (which I have not addressed here) about who benefits from the introduction of endocrine-disrupting chemicals into various environments. Clearly some businesses and individuals benefit from forms of polluting activities linked to endocrine-disrupting chemicals. As in the case of HRT, interests around endocrine-disrupting chemicals are part of both financial *and* sexual (bio)economies.

Sharing space with polar bears

The image of the polar bear is taken up throughout the multiple literatures on endocrine disruption. Like the OncoMouse™, but in substantially different ways (most significantly, polar bears represent contaminated nature that is produced unintentionally rather than through deliberate genetic modification), polar bears stand in for humans in technoscientific, popular science and environmentalist discourses. This is represented most clearly in the Cooperative Bank and WWF campaign in which humans begin to morph into polar bears. In their representative suffering, polar bears show that the 'natural order of things' is no longer as obvious as it seems – it is being mysteriously threatened in ways we humans are struggling to recognise. The 'natural' gaps between humans and animals and between certain groups of humans (English and Inuit, for example), have been breached by hormonal actions that demonstrate our shared vulnerabilities. WWF's (2000) characteristically pedagogic brochure, *Reducing Your Risk*, schematically represents this connection: cute, stylised line drawings accompanying text explaining 'Why be concerned?' represent a polar bear, a human baby and a frog all peering at the reader from a shared space. This is the shared space of contemporary technobiopower, in which the bodies and lives of humans and animals are situated within hormonal flows that exceed and disrupt boundaries of species, geography, generation and time, raising difficult new questions about suffering and whose responsibility it is to attempt to alleviate it.

Endocrine-disrupting chemicals present a significant challenge to how we think about sex hormones as messengers today. Invoking questions about bio-sociality and bodies, polar bears and polar-bear–human hybrids raise serious theoretical and ethopolitical issues for feminism. Feminist theories' diagnostic skills in analysing the folding of problematic histories of sex (Butler's 'burden of the sex of materiality') into contemporary discourse are valuable here, as are the resources provided by Haraway and those inspired by her[24] in framing questions about biological and cyborgian entities such as hormones and polar-bear–human hybrids.

---

[24] See, for example, Lykke 1996; Bryld 1996; Hird 2004; Braidotti 2006.

This work is just beginning, but will, as the rapidly multiplying literatures on global endocrine disruption indicate, become increasingly culturally significant. Discourses on endocrine disruptors provide challenges to feminist research on sex/gender and embodiment. As we respond to living in 'hormone-soaked' environments, bio-social embodiments will change, affecting what Grosz (1994: 187) calls 'the biological limits' that 'constrain' the body. Theoretical approaches to sex/gender and embodiment must develop to address such as yet unknowable embodied changes.

Conclusion: hormones as provocation

Despite their name, sex hormones are not currently very sexy. Compared to genes, chromosomes and stem cells, they seem rather old-fashioned biological actors. Unlike genes and stem cells, no major funding initiatives for the British social sciences focus on their actions. In many ways, hormones are quintessentially twentieth-century entities: 'born' in a time when scientific biology was very new, genetics hardly considered and stem cells only just 'discovered', they had their glory days in the mid to late century, gradually becoming mundane and even troublesome in more recent years. Hormonal action today is increasingly difficult to grasp as scientists and clinicians learn more about hormones, wonder about how even to define them as a group and raise serious questions about their safety as medications. Despite these difficulties, hormones have demonstrated great tenacity in remaining at the centre of explanations of 'life' and particularly of sex and sexual differences. In all kinds of discourses – technoscientific, biomedical, social scientific, popular, media – and in everyday conversation, hormones perform important explanatory work in descriptions of who we are and how we reproduce. They are active in bodies of all sorts; as endogenous chemicals, medications and environmental toxins. Sex hormones today surround us, affecting humans and other animals in barely perceptible ways, altering, it is claimed, what our futures might hold. Hormones and chemicals that act like them breach all kinds of boundaries: between species (creating polar-bear–human hybrids), places (the Arctic is suddenly near England), times (the effects of toxic chemicals are transgenerational) and sexes (males are demasculinised and feminised, females masculinised and defeminised). Human and other animal bodies are no longer hermetically sealed; they are open to hormonal global flows, to toxic chemical 'assaults', to invisible, long-term threats.

Sex hormones are also engaged in significant international (bio)economic flows, carrying particular understandings of bodies and sex in their global movements. These movements create significant connections between groups of humans and animals. The hormones composing the most popular HRT medication for women, for example, come from the urine of pregnant horses stabled in North America, creating complicated connections between women patients, manufacturers and the thousands of animals who suffer to produce this product. Although (until recently at least) these connections have proved vastly profitable for pharmaceutical companies, such profits are based on the promotion of HRT to particular groups of women, promotion that is framed by racist and classist exclusions. Other hormonal flows connect large numbers of relatively affluent women to small groups of unnamed, less affluent women. One of the most popular *in-vitro* fertilisation (IVF) drugs, for example, used by millions of women globally to stimulate their ovaries to produce multiple follicles for egg collection, is made from the urine of post-menopausal women living in one village in Argentina, collected and refined by Swiss pharmaceutical company Ferring.[1] Although referenced in the name of the drug – Menopur – these donating post*meno*pausal women remain almost invisible participants in global flows of hormone-related capital. Artificially produced sex hormones also produce vast profits for companies manufacturing various forms of contraceptive medication for women and, as in the case of male HRT, give rise to great hopes of profits for the company that will eventually produce an acceptable product for men (Oudshoorn 2003).

In all these forms, sex hormones from human and other animal bodies or chemically constituted in laboratories, create (bio)value and substantially alter bodies and lives.[2] Hormones taken as HRT, contraception or in infertility treatment change bodies in as-yet only partially understood ways. These changes may well affect others in connected environments: male fish in British rivers, for example, are showing signs of feminisation thought to be caused by the excretions of women contraceptive pill users (BBC News Online 2002). Especially if their effects are not limited to the individual person or generation, but can be passed on in sexual reproduction

---

[1] I was told this by a representative of the manufacturer at a conference in London, June 2006, but have not been able to find additional information about these women on the internet. These women are not paid to donate their urine: the representative was unsure, then, how they are 'incentivised' to participate in this process.

[2] For more detailed discussions, see Waldby (2002) who uses the term 'biovalue' and Franklin (2003) who uses the term 'biocapital formation' to describe the extraction of surplus value from biological materials.

(as in the DES case discussed in Chapter 6), hormones could still be described today, to borrow Barbara Seaman's emotive phrase, as 'the greatest experiment ever performed on women' (Seaman 2003).

The everyday familiarity of sex hormones obscures the sheer scale of this 'experiment'. Hormonal intervention in human and other animal reproduction dwarfs the levels of intervention currently undertaken in genetics, in the use of preimplantation genetic diagnosis (the so-called 'designer baby' technique) for example.[3] Hormones in the form of pills, patches, injections or implants remain the most popular contraceptive technology throughout the world. In terms of new reproductive technologies, whilst the implications of genetic technologies might be more newsworthy in their multiple connections to science-fiction scenarios, the use of sex hormones to stimulate the ovaries underpins almost all assisted conception, reprogenetic and human embryonic stem cell techniques.[4] It is not possible to perform IVF or preimplantation genetic diagnosis, or to create human embryonic stem cell lines, without eggs and eggs are not viably procured without hormonal ovarian stimulation. All of this contemporary biomedicine and technoscience, then, rides on the back of twentieth-century endocrinology: to use a biological metaphor, these reproductive and genetic technologies are nourished by the placenta of endocrinology. (Remember, as discussed in Chapter 2, the placenta is generated by both the mother and foetus, disrupting conventional distinctions between 'individuals'. Similarly, here, contemporary reproductive and genetic technologies both rely on and (re)create endocrinology.)

Sex hormones are excellent examples of Foucault's biopower and its second millennial counterpart, described by Donna Haraway (1997: 12) as technobiopower. As resilient twentieth-century actors underpinning much contemporary biomedicine and biological technoscience, hormones are a fascinating case study of the ways in which modern power takes hold of the body and of life itself. In his final chapter of *The History of Sexuality: an introduction*, Foucault (1987: 135–59) famously argues that biopower operates along two axes: one pertaining to populations and the other to individual bodies. Sex hormones are active along both axes. Firstly, as contraceptives and infertility drugs, hormones play important roles in literally creating and prohibiting populations. A paper presented

---

[3] For a social scientific analysis of this technique, see Roberts and Franklin 2005; Franklin and Roberts 2006.

[4] It is possible, although very rarely done (at least in Britain), to perform 'natural cycle' IVF in which hormones are not used to stimulate the ovaries. The First World Congress on Natural Cycle/Minimal Stimulation IVF was held in London in December 2006.

at the European Society of Human Reproduction and Embryology conference in June 2006, for example, argued that three free cycles of IVF
should be given to every infertile couple in Britain in order to stem the
problematically low birth rate (currently 1.8 births per woman) and the
consequently 'looming pensions crisis'. Rather than funding childcare
places or increasing immigration, hormone-stimulated reproduction is
promoted as an answer to these serious demographic issues: if IVF was
offered free to all infertile couples, a newspaper report states, 'the country would increase its population by 10,000 within two to three years'
(Sample 2006). The impact of such intervention is calculated to the
pound: the cost of each IVF baby is £12,931, meaning that the resultant
child's net lifetime contribution to the British economy would decrease
from £160,069 to £147,138. A loss worth bearing, author Professor Bill
Ledger, head of reproductive medicine at Sheffield University, argues.
Remaining uncalculated are the costs to women patients, to future
children, to other people, animals and the environment, of hormonal
stimulation and the other techniques of IVF. IVF figures here as a
neutral technology, not one causing serious psychosocial distress
(Throsby 2005) or that involves as yet unclear physical implications for
patients, their offspring and their environments.

Hormones also modify or 'discipline' individual bodies. Pharmaceutical
companies promote HRT as creating 'liberation' for the contemporary
cohort of late-middle-aged women and men, 'freeing' them to continue
their economically productive and psychologically fulfilling lives. Rather
than challenging cultural ageism or altering entrenched patterns of obses-
sive overwork, sex hormones are figured (and swallowed) as the solution to
individuals' difficulties in keeping up with life in contemporary capitalist
cultures. Again (although the media and popular books have given some
airplay to these concerns) the potential long-term effects of such interventions are usually left aside in these discourses.

In a recent literature review, anthropologist Linda Hogle (2005) analyses social scientific work on enhancement technologies (cosmetic surgery,
psychopharmaceuticals, new reproductive and genetic technologies and
prosthetics), suggesting that the promotion of biomedical 'solutions' to
significant social and cultural problems is endemic in contemporary western countries. The strong level of interest in and support for the development of enhancement technologies, she argues, 'indicates the kinds of
decisions being made about the appropriateness of using biology to solve
social problems such as aging, fairness and inequality of opportunity, and
care of the self' (Hogle 2005: 696). Bodily enhancements, although linked

to the rise of late twentieth-century consumer culture, cannot be explained solely as commodification processes. 'Enhancements', Hogle writes, 'are upgrades. Upgrades support scientific research agendas and the ongoing production of goods and services that suit the needs of global exchanges'. 'At the same time', she adds, 'the ability to engineer bodily functions gives currency to the illusion of controlling predictability in an unpredictable world' (Hogle 2005: 703–4). From the perspectives of contemporary bio-power, many social problems are too hard to fix, so bodies become a good substitute for something both experts and laypeople/consumers *can* do something about. 'In the emerging ethics of enhancement technologies', Hogle surmises, 'bodies made to be reliant, more enduring, and attractive will be prepared for any contingency of social life, labor, or global condition' (Hogle 2005: 704). Late capitalism, in other words, creates unsolvably complex problems for social life, but (techno)biopower can at least (attempt to) make bodies that are better able to deal with its demands.

For Foucault, sex is the pivotal point between the two axes of biopower: 'Broadly speaking', he writes, 'at the juncture of "the body" and the "population," sex became a crucial target of a power organized around the management of life rather than the menace of death' (Foucault 1987: 147). Sex, in this analysis, is connected to life, representing power's shift away from violent destruction to the facilitation of kinds of life or vitality. As in the case of sex hormones, 'sex' concerns materiality and vitality, bodies and life itself. This connection between sex and vitality is of enduring interest to feminist theory.

Feminism and vital material bodies

The overarching project of *Messengers of Sex* has been to bring social scientific and cultural studies work on technoscience and biomedicine into dialogue with contemporary feminist theories of the body.[5] This book has

---

[5] In *Transpositions*, Braidotti (2006) argues that one of the major axes of discursive segregation in contemporary thought is that between science studies and what she calls 'philosophies of the subject' (feminist and otherwise). 'The missing links of this dialogue', she argues, 'are manifold and they converge on a collision course upon the theme of "posthumanism". If such a theme is to strike a note of resonance and relevance in both communities', she contends, 'it needs more detailed analyses than have been offered so far. Science studies need to address their resistance to theories of the subject, and to notions such as embodiment and affectivity. Philosophies of the subject, on the other hand, have to confront their mistrust and mis-cognition of bio-sciences' (Braidotti 2006: 138). I agree with Braidotti on this point and hope that this book goes some way to build these 'missing links'.

introduced several feminist concepts addressing bodily sexual differences
including performativity, articulation, interimplication and embodiment.
All of these concepts figure bodies as neither entirely biological nor entirely
social, but as entities confounding this distinction. Judith Butler's (1990,
1993) term 'performativity' is perhaps the best-known in contemporary
feminist theory. As outlined in the Introduction, this concept usefully
describes a temporally situated process of materialisation of sexed/gen-
dered bodies, but privileges language and discourse as the active elements
in this process. Elizabeth Grosz (1994) focuses more explicitly on the
potentiality of the biological, deploying the metaphor of the Möbius
strip (an inverted figure eight) to represent the undecidable flow between
the (biological) inside and the (social) outside of bodies. She describes the
biological and the social as 'interimplicated': a term that has been useful
here in thinking about the relations between hormones and human and
non-human social actors.

Haraway (1997) uses the term 'articulation' to describe the relation
between 'nature' and 'culture'. Articulation replaces 'representation' as a
description of what scientists do when they engage with nature, figuring
nature or the world itself (bodies, animals, cells, genes, hormones, gels,
test tubes, etc.) as active in such engagements. Technoscience, in the
articulation model, is a social relationship between a variety of actors:
bodies are social and always in relation to other entities. What is political,
then, is how these relationships get done, by whom and at what costs.
Feminism, Haraway suggests, has much to contribute to articulating and
beginning to answer these questions. Questions about the OncoMouse^{TM}
provide an excellent example. Feminists need to be involved in calculations made about the value of human and other animal lives lived with and
without breast cancer, and how much money and time should be spent
working on animals like OncoMouse^{TM} to develop knowledge about
oncological processes and treatments. In Chapter 6, I discussed polar-
bear–human hybrids as 'cousins' to OncoMouse^{TM}, suggesting that in this
similar case Haraway's questions about suffering provide more useful
avenues for thought than the nostalgic concerns of environmentalist
organisations and popular scientific literature. Rosi Braidotti elaborates
a related argument in Deleuzian terms, talking about 'sustainability'
rather than suffering. For her, 'ethics is related to the physics and biology
of bodies. This means', she explains, 'that it deals with the question of
what exactly a body can do and how much it can take' (Braidotti 2006:
129). As for Haraway, the fundamentals here are not about 'nature' or
'purity' but about bodily potentials and relationality; what Deleuze and

Guattari call 'becomings'. For Braidotti and for Haraway, these questions of suffering or sustainability are questions for collective, political consideration; consideration that takes issues of sex/gender into serious account. 'The limits of what a body can do', Braidotti writes,

> need to be experimented with collectively, so as to produce effective cartographies of how much bodies can take, or thresholds of sustainability. They also aim to create collective bonds, a new affective community or polity. This must include an evaluation of the costs involved in pursuing active processes of change and of recognition of the pain and the difficulty these entail.
>
> *(Braidotti 2006: 227–8)*

The material forms of this collectivity remain nebulous in Braidotti's account, but in the case of sex hormones, it is important that questions of 'how much bodies can take' do not remain in the realms of technoscience and biomedicine alone. The answers to these questions must be bio-social and psycho-social: biomedicine's and technoscience's drive is often to push bodies to extremes (to use ovarian-stimulating hormones to produce as many follicles as possible in an IVF cycle, for example; or to use HRT to 'eliminate' aging) without paying serious attention to the multiple, complex costs of such activities. *Messengers of Sex* elaborates how such costs might be thought of in feminist terms and brings these issues to the attention of a community of feminist scholars and activists.

The biosciences *are* becoming increasingly important to feminist theorists today, with a number of well-known philosophers producing books dealing specifically with biology in the last few years. As described in the Introduction, in the Deleuze-inspired works of Braidotti and Grosz, biology is understood as a positive force, something that is enabling, productive, provocative.[6] Grosz calls this force 'nature', whilst Braidotti refers to *zoe*, 'the surplus vitality of living matter' (Braidotti 2006: 47).[7] In their work, this vitality or force lines up somewhat problematically with what is described and produced in technoscience and biomedicine as 'biology'. In places in Grosz's work, this alignment is strong (in her discussion of Darwin's theories, for example); elsewhere, technoscience and biomedicine disappear altogether. In Braidotti's *Transpositions*, the term *bios* holds a place for the entities articulated by technoscience, but the distinction

---

[6] Grosz (2006: 51) uses the term provocation to describe nature's relation to culture: 'In other words', she writes, 'nature bequeaths to all the forms of culture a series of problems or provocations ... which each cultural form must address, in its own way, even if it cannot solve them.'

[7] Others also use the terms 'vitality' and 'vital materialism'. See, for example, Hird 2004; Fraser, Kember and Lury 2005.

between *zoe* and *bios* tends to collapse (she often uses the conjoined term *zoe/bios* in talking about bodies). This collapse is inevitable: the attempt to hold open a space of pure vitality, of a biological or life force outside of technoscience or biomedicine is unsustainable (see also Fraser *et al.* 2005: 6). Spivak's (1994: 177) remark – 'The body, like all other things, cannot be thought as such. Like all other things I have never tried to approach the body as such' – is highly relevant here. How would it be possible to think or speak of a vital force 'as such', outside technoscience and biomedicine? As soon as we move away from generalities ('the body', 'nature', '*zoe*') towards specificities such as sex hormones, we are in a world constituted by practices, histories, meanings and power relations, that is, technoscience and biomedicine. This is *not* to say that there is no vital force or positivity of the kind described by Braidotti and Grosz – indeed the point of this book has been to argue that hormones arguably constitute such a force – but rather that as soon as we start to think or speak about them, we engage technoscientific or biomedical discourses and thus immediately become entwined in problematic inheritances. The difficulty for feminist science studies, then, is how to theorise the activity of biological actors such as hormones without uncritically aligning with technoscience.[8]

Perhaps the most common textual strategy for dealing with this dilemma, employed by both Braidotti and Haraway, is the propagation of conjoined neologisms. This joining of unlikely pairs is ubiquitous in contemporary social science and humanities research on technoscience and biomedicine. In this book I have cited, for example, *zoe/bios*, material-semiotic, naturecultures, biopower, technobiopower, sex/gender, bio-sociality, biovalue, and my personal favourite, bio-social. All of these phrases signal the disruption of modern conceptual dichotomies: between nature and culture, the biological and the social. Importantly, however, in maintaining the original words in these neologisms, social theorists signal that what is at stake is *not* the complete disintegration or breakdown of categories, but rather the reconfiguring of boundaries and the visibility

---

[8] These issues are discussed further in an article co-written with Adrian Mackenzie (Roberts and Mackenzie 2006). Much humanities and social science work on science, we suggest, can be classified as either critical or affirmative of technoscience. A third, much smaller and more recent group, demonstrates a new attitude that we characterise as 'experimental'. This attitude openly engages with technoscientific concepts and practices, putting these to surprising ends by approaching them in a spirit eschewing both condemnation and celebration.

of new movements, mobilities or flows across them.[9] The concept of messaging highlights this movement, describing hormonal action as flows across 'the social' and 'the biological'; flows that are generative of historically specific materialisations of what we understand of these two 'categories'. Hormones, in other words, are radically relational: as messengers of sex, they work with other entities to enact sex as a set of contingent, yet impressively enduring, relations.

Ernest Starling's choice of the classical Greek word *hormao* to form the root of the modern scientific term 'hormone' was felicitous. Etymologically, *hormao* means to excite or provoke. These are interesting actions: to provoke is to set something off, rather than to control or produce it. There is an openness in this verb that leaves space for relations other than determinism. As provocative messengers, hormones create relations in articulation with other actors, retaining the potential to enact other relations in other times and spaces. Hormones are thus inherently (bio)political; their actions provoke complex and profound questions about what kinds of bodies live and what kinds of lives we hope for.

Over the last one hundred years, endogenous and exogenous sex hormones have been enrolled with humans and non-humans to explain, justify and facilitate certain bodies and behaviours. These bodies and behaviours have been described as 'sex' and are widely understood as natural or biological and consequently as desirable and even unchangeable. In the second half of the last century, vast quantities of sex hormones entered our lives as human-made products and will continue to do so in the foreseeable future with as-yet unknowable effects. It is time, then, to radically retheorise their messaging actions and to experiment with articulating with sex hormones in ways that cause less suffering for humans and other animals and that open onto living with multiple forms of difference.

---

[9] A number of social theorists have recently used these terms: see, for example, Urry (2003) who writes about global flows and mobilities and Mol and Law (1994) who describe anemias as fluids.

References

Adami, Hans-Olav and Persson, Ingemar. 1995. Hormone Replacement Therapy and Cancer: A remaining controversy? *Journal of the American Medical Association* 274(2): 178–9

Akrich, Madeleine. 1992. The De-Scription of Technical Objects. In W. E. Bijker and J. Law (eds.), *Shaping Technology, Building Society: Studies in socio-technical change*, pp. 205–44. Cambridge, MA: MIT Press

Alonso, L. C. and Rosenfield, R. L. 2002. Oestrogens and Puberty. *Best Practice in Research in Clinical Endocrinology and Metabolism* 16(1): 13–30

Amsterdamska, Olga. 1990. Surely You Are Joking Monsieur Latour! *Science, Technology and Human Values* 15(4): 495–504

Anway, Matthew D., Cupp, Andrea S., Uzumcu, Mehmet and Skinner, Michael K. 2005. Epigenetic Transgenerational Actions of Endocrine Disruptors and Male Fertility. *Science* 3 June: 1466–9

Arnold, Arthur, P. and Breedlove, S. Marc. 1985. Organizational and Activational Effects of Sex Steroids on Brain and Behavior: A reanalysis. *Hormones and Behavior* 19: 469–98

Atkins, Lucy. 2004. Throw Out the Bath Water? *Chemical World Supplement, The Guardian,* May 8: 20–3

Avila, D. M., Zoppi, S. and McPhaul, M. J. 2001. The Androgen Receptor (AR) in Syndromes of Androgen Insensitivity and in Prostate Cancer. *Journal of Steroid Biochemistry and Molecular Biology* 76(1–5): 135–42

Avis, N. E., Crawford, S., Stellato, R. and Longcop, C. 2001. Longitudinal Study of Hormone Levels and Depression among Women Transitioning Through Menopause. *Climacteric* 4(3): 243–9

Bain, J. 2001. Andropause: Testosterone replacement therapy for aging men. *Canadian Family Physician* 47: 91–7

Baker, Susan W. 1980. Biological Influences on Human Sex and Gender. *Signs: Journal of Women in Culture and Society* 6(1): 80–96

Balsamo, Anne. 1996. *Technologies of the Gendered Body: Reading cyborg women.* Durham, NC and London: Duke University Press

Baron-Cohen, Simon 2004. *The Essential Difference.* London: Penguin Books

Baron-Cohen, Simon, Lutchmaya, Svetlana and Knickmeyer, Rebecca. 2004. *Prenatal Testosterone in Mind: Amniotic fluid studies.* Cambridge, MA and London: MIT Press

BBC News Online. 2002. River Pollution Sparks Fertility Fears. www.bbc.co.uk/1/hi/uk/1877162.stm. 17 March. Last accessed 25 September 2006

Beach, Frank A. 1975. Behavioral Endocrinology: An emerging discipline. *American Scientist* 63, March–April: 178–87

Beauvoir, Simone de. 1988 [1949]. *The Second Sex.* H. M. Parshley (trans. and ed.). London: Pan Books

Bell, Susan. 1987. Changing Ideas: The medicalization of menopause. *Social Science and Medicine* 24(6): 535–42

Beral V. and Million Women Study Collaborators. 2003. Breast Cancer and Hormone-Replacement Therapy in the Million Women Study. *Lancet* 362: 419–27

Berger, Maurice, Wallis, Brian and Watson, Simon (eds.). 1995. *Constructing Masculinity.* New York and London: Routledge

Berglund, Hans, Lindström, Per and Savic, Ivanka. 2006. Brain Response to Putative Pheromones in Lesbian Women. *Proceedings of the National Academy of Sciences* 103(21): 8269–74

Berkson, D. Lindsey. 2000. *Hormone Deception: How everyday foods and products are disrupting your hormones – and how to protect yourself and your family.* New York: Contemporary Books

Bhavnani, Kum-Kum and Haraway, Donna. 1994. Shifting the Subject: A conversation between Kum-Kum Bhavnani and Donna Haraway, 12 April 1993, Santa Cruz, California. Justine Meyers (transcriber). *Feminism and Psychology* 4(1):19–39

Biddulph, Steven. 1997. *Raising Boys: Why boys are different – and how to help them become happy and well-balanced men.* London: Thorsons

Bimonte, Heather A., Fitch, R. Holly and Denenberg, Victor H. 2000. Neonatal Estrogen Blockage Prevents Normal Callosal Responsiveness to Estradiol in Adulthood. *Developmental Brain Research* 122(2): 149–55

Birke, Lynda. 2000. Sitting on the Fence: Biology, feminism and gender-bending environments. *Women's Studies International Forum* 23(5): 587–99

1999. *Feminism and the Biological Body.* Edinburgh University Press

Birke, Lynda I. A. and Sadler, Dawn. 1985. Maternal Behavior in Rats and the Effects of Neonatal Progestins Given to Pups. *Developmental Psychobiology* 18(6): 467–75

Bland, Lucy. 1995. *Banishing the Beast: English Feminism and sexual morality 1885–1914.* London: Penguin Books

Bleier, Ruth. 1984. *Science and Gender.* Elmsford, NY: Pergamon

Bordo, Susan. 1993. *Unbearable Weight: Feminism, western culture, and the body.* Berkeley, LA and London: University of California Press

Borell, Merriley. 1976. Organotherapy, British Physiology, and the Discovery of the Internal Secretions. *Journal of the History of Biology* 9(2): 235–68

1985. Organotherapy and the Emergence of Reproductive Endocrinology. *Journal of the History of Biology* 18(1): 1–30

1987. Biologists and the Promotion of Birth Control Research, 1918–1938. *Journal of the History of Biology* 20(1): 51–87

Boulet, M.J., Oddens, B.J., Lehert, P., Vemer, H.M. and Visser, A. 1994. Climacteric and Menopause in Seven South-East Asian Countries. *Maturitas* 19(3): 155–6

Bradshaw, John and Rogers, Lesley J. 1993. *The Evolution of Lateral Asymmetries, Language, Tool Use and Intellect*. San Diego, CA: Academic Press

Braidotti, Rosi. 1989. The Politics of Ontological Difference. In Teresa Brennan (ed.), *Between Feminism and Psychoanalysis*, pp. 89–105. London: Routledge

2002. *Metamorphoses: Towards a materialist theory of becoming*, Cambridge: Polity

2006. *Transpositions: On nomadic ethics*, Cambridge and Malden, MA: Polity

Brennan, Teresa. 2004. *The Transmission of Affect*. Ithaca and London: Cornell University Press

Brinton, L.A. and Schairer, C. 1993. Estrogen Replacement Therapy and Breast Cancer Risk. *Epidemiologic Reviews* 15(1): 66–79

Bryld, Mette. 1996. Dialogues with Dolphins and Other Extraterrestrials: Displacements in gendered space. In Nina Lykke and Rosi Braidotti (eds.), *Between Monsters, Goddesses and Cyborgs: Feminist confrontations with science, medicine and cyberspace*, pp. 47–71. London: Zed Books

Bunkle, Phillida. 1997. Calling the Shots? The international politics of depo-provera. In Sandra Harding (ed.), *The 'Racial' Economy of Science: Toward a democratic future*, pp. 287–302. Bloomington and Indianapolis: Indiana University Press

Burkeman, Oliver. 2002. HRT Study Cancelled over Cancer and Stroke Fears. *The Guardian*, 10 July. http://education.guardian.co.uk/higher/medicalscience/ story/0,,752653,00.html Last accessed 25 September 2006

Burr, Chandler. 1993. Homosexuality and Biology. *The Atlantic Monthly* 271(3): 47–65

Butler, Judith. 1990. *Gender Trouble: Feminism and the subversion of identity*. New York and London: Routledge

1993. *Bodies that Matter: On the discursive limits of 'sex'*. New York and London: Routledge

1994. Against Proper Objects. *Differences: A Journal of Feminist Cultural Studies* 6(2–3): 1–26

2004. *Undoing Gender*. New York and London: Routledge

Byne, William, Lasco, Mitchell S., Kemether, Eileen, Shinwari, Akbar, Edgar, Mark A., Morgello, Susan, Jones, Liesl B. and Tobet, Stuart. 2000. The Interstitial Nuclei of the Human Anterior Hypothalamus: An investigation of sexual variation in volume and cell size, number and density. *Brain Research* 856(1–2): 254–8

Byne, William, Tobet, Stuart, Mattiace, Linda A., Lasco, Mitchell S., Kemether, Eileen, Edgar, Mark A., Morgello, Susan, Buschbaum, Monte S. and Jones, Liesl B. 2001. The Interstitial Nuclei of the Human Anterior Hypothalamus: An investigation of variation with sex, sexual orientation, and HIV status. *Hormones and Behavior* 40: 86–92

Cadbury, Deborah. 1998. *The Feminization of Nature: Our future at risk*. London: Penguin Books

Caine, Barbara. 1992. *Victorian Feminists*. Oxford University Press

Callon, Michel. 1986. Some Elements of a Sociology of Translation: Domestication of the scallops and the fishermen of St. Brieuc Bay. In J. Law (ed.), *Power, Action and Belief*, pp. 196–233. London: Routledge and Kegan Paul

Callon, Michel and Rabeharisoa, Vollona. 2004. Gino's Lesson on Humanity: Genetics, mutual entanglements and the sociologist's role. *Economy and Society* 33(1): 1–27

Canguilhem, Georges. 1988. *Ideology and Rationality in the History of the Life Sciences*. Arthur Goldhammer (trans.). Cambridge, MA: MIT Press

  1994. *The Vital Rationalist: Selected writings from Georges Canguilhem*. François Delaporte (trans.). New York: Zone Books

Capezuti, Elizabeth, Strumpf, Neville E., Lois, K., Grisso, Jeane Ann and Maislin, Greg. 1998. The Relationship Between Physical Restraint Removal and Falls and Injuries among Nursing Home Residents. *Journal of Gerontology* 53A(1): 47–52

Carlson, Neil R. 1992. *Foundations of Physiological Psychology*, 2nd edn. Boston: Allyn and Bacon

Carson, Rachel. 1962. *Silent Spring*. London: Hamish Hamilton

Carter, C. Sue and Getz, Lowell L. 1993. Monogamy and the Prairie Vole. *Scientific American* June: 70–6

Chase, Cheryl. 1998a. Hermaphrodites with Attitude: Mapping the emergence of intersex political activism. *GLQ: A Journal of Lesbian and Gay Studies* 4(2): 189–211

  1998b. Surgical Progress Is Not the Answer to Intersexuality. *Journal of Clinical Ethics* 9(4): 385–92

  1999. Rethinking Treatment for Ambiguous Genitalia. *Pediatric Nursing* 25: 451–5

Cheah, Pheng. 1996. Mattering. *Diacritics* 26(1): 108–39

Cilag. 1995. Evorel® advertisement 1. *British Journal of Sexual Medicine* 22(1): 28

  1996. Evorel® advertisement 2. *British Journal of Sexual Medicine* 23(1): 8

Clarke, Adele. 1998. *Disciplining Reproduction*. Berkeley, LA and London: University of California Press

Clarke, Adele E. and Fujimura, Joan (eds.). 1992. *The Right Tools for the Job: At work in twentieth-century life*. Princeton University Press

Cobb, Ivo Geike. 1935. *The Glands of Destiny (A Study of the Personality)*, 2nd edn. London: William Heineman (Medical Books)

Cobbs, Elizabeth R. and Ralapati, Anuradha N. 1998. Health of Older Women. *Medical Clinics of North America* 82(1): 127–44

Colborn, Theo, Dumanoski, Dianne and Peterson, John. 1996. *Our Stolen Future: Are we threatening our fertility, intelligence and survivial – A scientific detective story*. London: Little, Brown and Company

Coney, Sandra. 1991. *The Menopause Industry: A guide to medicine's 'discovery' of the midlife woman*. Melbourne: Spinifex Press

Connell, R. W. 2000. *The Men and the Boys*. Sydney: Allen and Unwin

Conrad, Peter and Gabe, Jonathon. 1999. *Sociological Perspectives on the New Genetics*. Oxford: Blackwell Publishers

Co-operative Bank and World Wildlife Fund. 2004. Polar Bears Don't Live in Houses Campaign. *The Guardian Weekend* 15 May: 50

Cowlishaw, Gillian. 1982. Family Planning: A post-contact problem. In Janice
    Reid (ed.), *Health and Healing in Aboriginal Society*, pp. 31–48. St Lucia:
    University of Queensland Press
Crews, David. 1988. The Problem with Gender. *Psychobiology* 16(4): 321–34
    1994. Animal Sexuality. *Scientific American* 270(1): 96–103
Curtis, Polly. 2004. Finger Points to Good Research Skills. *The Guardian*,
    20 October
Davidson, Nancy. 1995. Hormone-Replacement Therapy: Breast versus heart
    versus bone. *New England Journal of Medicine* 332(4): 1638–9
Davis, Kathy. 1995. *Reshaping the Female Body: The dilemma of cosmetic surgery*.
    London and New York: Routledge
De Bendern, Paul. 2002. Toxins Put Arctic Polar Bears and Humans at Risk. *World
    Environment News*, Reuters, www.planetark.org., 3 October. Last accessed
    27 July 2003
Dennerstein, Lorraine. 1993/34. The Controversial Menopause. *21C: The
    Magazine of the Australian Commission for the Future*, Summer: 12–17
Doell, Ruth G. and Longino, Helen E. 1988. Sex Hormones and Human
    Behaviour: A critique of the linear model. *Journal of Homosexuality* 15(3/4):
    55–78
Donovan, Bernard. 1988. *Humors, Hormones and the Mind: An approach to the
    understanding of behaviour*. New York: Stockton Press
Dorey, Catherine N. (2003) *Chemical Legacy: Contamination of the child*. London:
    Greenpeace
Doyal, Lesley. 1995. *What Makes Women Sick? Gender and the political economy of
    health*. London: Macmillan Press
Duden, Barbara. 1991. *The Woman Beneath the Skin: A doctor's patients in
    eighteenth-century Germany*. Thomas Dunlap (trans.). Cambridge, MA and
    London: Harvard University Press
    1993. *Disembodying Women: Perspectives on pregnancy and the unborn*. Lee
    Hoinacki (trans.). Cambridge, MA: Harvard University Press
Dumit, Joseph. 2002. Drugs for Life. *Molecular Interventions* 2(3): 124–7
    2004. *Picturing Personhood: Brain scans and biomedical identity*. Princeton
    University Press
    2005. The Depsychiatrisation of Mental Illness. *Journal of Public Mental Health*
    4(3): 8–13
Edwards, J., Franklin, S., Hirsch, E., Price and Strathern, M. 1999. *Technologies of
    Procreation: Kinship in the age of assisted conception*, 2nd edn (with additional
    material). London: Routledge
Ehrhardt, Anke A. 1984. Gender Differences: A biosocial perspective. *Nebraska
    Symposium on Motivation* 33: 37–57
Ehrhardt, Anke, A. and Meyer-Balhburg, Heino F. L. 1981. Effects of Prenatal Sex
    Hormones on Gender-Related Behavior. *Science* 211: 1312–18
Ellerington, M. C., Whitcroft, S. I. T. and Whitehead, M. I. 1992. HRT
    Developments in Therapy. *British Medical Bulletin* 48(2): 401–25
Elwyn, Glynn, Edwards, Adrian, Gwyn, Richard and Grol, Richard. 1999.
    Towards a Feasible Model for Shared Decision-making: Focus group study
    with general practitioners. *British Medical Journal* 319: 753–6

Ettinger, Bruce. 1998. Overview of Estrogen Replacement Therapy: A historical perspective. *Proceedings of the Society for Experimental Biology and Medicine* 217(1): 2–5

European Environmental Bureau, EPHA Environmental Network, Friends of the Earth Europe, Greenpeace International, WWF and Women in Europe for a Common Future. 2005. NGOs' Five Key Demands to Improve REACH. www.foeeurope.org/safer_chemicals/five_key_demands.pdf. Last accessed 25 September 2006

European HRT-Network Foundation and Contraception Study Group. 2001. *Practical HRT.* www.hrtnet.org/prachrt/toc.htm. Last accessed 10 October 2003

Farrell, Elizabeth. 2003. Medical Choices Available for Management of Menopause. *Best Practice and Research in Clinical Endocrinology and Metabolism* 17(1): 1–6

Fausto-Sterling, Anne. 1992. *Myths of Gender: Biological theories about women and men.* Revised edn. New York: Basic Books

1993. The Five Sexes: Why male and female are not enough. *The Sciences* March/April: 20–5

1995. How to Build a Man. In Maurice Berger, Brian Wallis and Simon Watson (eds.), *Constructing Masculinity*, pp. 127–34. New York and London: Routledge

2000. *Sexing the Body: Gender politics and the construction of sexuality.* New York: Basic Books

Ferguson, Sherry A. 2002. Effects on Brain and Behavior Caused by Developmental Exposure to Endocrine Disruptors with Estrogenic Effects. *Neurotoxicology and Teratology* 24: 1–3

Fernald, Russell, D. 1993. Cichlids in Love: What a fish's social caste tells the fish's brain about sex. *The Sciences* July/August: 27–31

Finkler, Kaja. 2000. *Experiencing the New Genetics: Family and kinship on the medical frontier.* Philadelphia: University of Pennsylvania Press

Finnegan, Judy. 2002. HRT is a Change for the Better. *Daily Express*, Saturday, 1 May: 15

Fitch, R. H., Cowell, P. E. and Denenberg, V. H. 1998. The Female Phenotype: Nature's default? *Developmental Neuropsychology* 14(2/3): 213–31

Fitch, R. H. and Denenberg, V. H. 1998. A Role for Ovarian Hormones in Sexual Differentiation of the Brain. *Behavioral and Brain Sciences* 21(3): 311–35

Fletcher, Suzanne W. and Colditz, Graham A. 2002. Failure of Estrogen Plus Progestin Therapy for Prevention. *Journal of the American Medical Association* 288(3): 1–6

Foucault, Michel. 1987. *The History of Sexuality: An introduction.* Robert Hurley (trans.). London: Penguin Books

1988. *Madness and Civilization: A history of insanity in the Age of Reason.* New York: Vintage

1994. *The Birth of the Clinic: An archeology of medical perception.* Reprint edn. New York: Vintage

1995. *Discipline and Punish: The birth of the prison.* Reprint edn. New York: Vintage

Fox, Helen E., Stephanie A. White, Kao, Mimi H. and Fernald, D. 1997. Stress and Dominance in a Social Fish. *Journal of Neuroscience* 17(16): 6463–9

Francis, Richard C., Soma, Kiran and Fernald, Russell D. 1993. Social Regulation of the Brain-Pituitary-Gonadal Axis. *Proceedings of the National Academy of Science USA* 90 (August): 7794–8

Franklin, Sarah. 2001. Culturing Biology: Cell lines for the second millennium. *Health* 5(3): 321–40

2003. Ethical Biocapital: New strategies of stem cell culture. In Sarah Franklin and Margaret Lock (eds.), *Remaking Life and Death: Toward an anthropology of the biosciences*, pp. 97–127. Sante Fe and Oxford: School of American Research Press

Franklin, Sarah and McKinnon, Susan (eds.). 2003. *Relative Values: Reconfiguring kinship studies*. Durham, NC and London: Duke University Press

Franklin, Sarah and Roberts, Celia. 2006. *Born and Made: An ethnography of preimplantation genetic diagnosis*. Princeton University Press

Fraser, Mariam, Kember, Sarah and Lury, Celia. 2005. Inventive Life: Approaches to the new vitalism. *Theory, Culture and Society* 22(1): 1–14

Fraser, Suzanne. 2003. *Cosmetic Surgery, Gender and Culture*. London: Palgrave.

Friends of the Earth. 2001a. *Chemicals in the Home: A parent's guide*. London: Friends of the Earth with support from the National Childbirth Trust.

2001b. *Fact Sheet: Chemicals and Breastmilk*. www.foe.co.uk/resource/factsheets/chemicals_breastmilk.pdf. Last accessed 25 September 2006

2001c. *Press Briefing: Chemicals and health*. www.foe.co.uk/resource/briefings/chemicals_and_health.pdf. Last accessed 25 September 2006

2001d. *Chemicals and Your Health: Briefing*. www.foe.co.uk/campaigns/safer_chemicals. Last accessed 25 September 2006

Frith, Maxine. 2003. Revealed: HRT causes breast cancer in 2,000 women in a year. *The Independent* 8 August: 1

Fujimura, Joan H. 1996. *Crafting Science: A sociohistory of the quest for the genetics of cancer*. Cambridge, MA: Harvard University Press

2006. 'Sex Genes': A critical sociomaterial approach to the politics and molecular genetics of sex determination. *Signs: A journal of women in society and culture* 32(1)

Fuss, Diana. 1994. Reading like a Feminist. In Naomi Schor and Elizabeth Weed (eds.), *The Essential Difference*, pp. 98–115. Bloomington and Indianapolis: Indiana University Press

Gallagher, Catherine and Laqueur, Thomas (eds.). 1987. *The Making of the Modern Body: Sexuality and society in the nineteenth century*. Berkeley, LA and London: University of California Press

Gatens, Moira. 1983. A Critique of the Sex/Gender Distinction. In Judith Allen and Paul Patton (eds.), *Beyond Marxism: Interventions after Marx*, pp. 143–60. Sydney: Intervention Press

1996. *Imaginary Bodies: Ethics, embodiment and corporeality*. New York and London: Routledge

Gilman, Sander L. 1985. Damaged Men: Thoughts on Kafka's body. In Maurice Berger, Brian Wallis and Simon Watson (eds.), *Constructing Masculinity*, pp. 176–89. New York and London: Routledge

1991. *The Jew's Body*. New York: Routledge

1993. *Freud, Race and Gender*. Princeton University Press

1995. *Picturing Health and Illness: Images of identity and difference*. Baltimore: Johns Hopkins University Press

Gorman, Christine. 1992. Sizing Up the Sexes. *Time Australia*, 20 January (3): 30–7

Gould, Stephen Jay. 1993. American Polygeny and Craniometry Before Darwin: Blacks and Indians as separate, inferior species. In Sandra Harding (ed.), *The 'Racial' Economy of Science: Toward a democratic future*, pp. 84–115. Bloomington and Indianapolis: Indiana University Press

Greenpeace. 2003. *Human Impacts of Man-Made Chemicals*. Greenpeace: London, October

2005. *Poisoning the Unborn*, 8 September. www.greenpeace.org/international/news/poisoning-the-unborn111. Last accessed 25 September 2006

Greer, Germaine. 1991. *The Change: Women, aging and the menopause*. London: Hamish Hamilton

Gregory, Jennie. 1935. *ABC of the Endocrines*. Baltimore: The Williams and Wilkins Company

Griffiths, Frances. 1999. Women's Control and Choice Regarding HRT. *Social Science and Medicine* 49: 469–81

Grosz, Elizabeth. 1989. *Sexual Subversions: Three French feminists*. Sydney: Allen and Unwin

1990. A Note on Essentialism and Difference. In Sneja Gunew (ed.), *Feminist Knowledge: Critique and construct*, pp. 332–44. New York: Routledge

1994. *Volatile Bodies: Toward a corporeal feminism*. Sydney: Allen and Unwin

1999. Darwin and Feminism: Preliminary investigations for a possible alliance. *Australian Feminist Studies* 14(29): 31–45

2005. *Time Travels: Feminism, nature, power*. Durham, NC and London: Duke University Press

Guillemin, Marilys. 2000a. Blood, Bone, Women and HRT: Co-construction in the menopause clinic. *Australian Feminist Studies* 15(32): 191–203

2000b. Working Practices of the Menopause Clinic. *Science, Technology and Human Values* 25(4): 448–70

Gullette, Margaret Morganroth. 1994. All Together Now: The new sexual politics of midlife bodies. In Laurence Goldstein (ed.), *The Male Body*, pp. 221–47. Ann Arbor: Michigan University Press

1997. Menopause as a Magic Marker: Discursive consolidation in the United States and strategies for cultural combat. In P. Komesaroff, P. Rothfield and J. Daly (eds.), *Reinterpreting Menopause: Cultural and philosophical issues*, pp. 176–99. New York and London: Routledge

2004. *Aged by Culture*. University of Chicago Press

Gunew, Sneja and Yeatman, Anna. 1995. *Feminism and the Politics of Difference*. Sydney: Allen and Unwin

Haeberle, Erwin J. 1981. Swastika, Pink Triangle and Yellow Star: The destruction of sexology and the persecution of homosexuals in Nazi Germany. *Journal of Sex Research* 17(3): 270–87

Hall, Diana Long. 1976a. Biology, Sex Hormones and Sexism in the 1920s. In M. Wartofsky and C. Could (eds.), *Women and Philosophy: Toward a theory of liberation*, pp. 81–96. New York: G. P. Putnam's Press

1976b. The Critic and the Advocate: Contrasting British views on the state of endocrinology in the early 1920s. *Journal of the History of Biology* 9(2): 269–85

Hamilton, David. 1986. *The Monkey Gland Affair*. London: Chatto and Windus

Hammonds, Evelynn. 1994. Black (W)holes and the Geometry of Black Feminist Sexuality. *Differences: A journal of feminist cultural studies* 6(2–3): 126–45

Haraway, Donna J. 1978. Animal Sociology and a Natural Economy of the Body Politic, Part I: A politic physiology of dominance; and Part II: The Past is the Contested Zone: Human nature and theories of production and reproduction in primate behavior. *Signs: A Journal of Women in Culture and Society* 4(1): 21–36 and 37–60

1989. *Primate Visions: Gender, race and nature in the world of modern science*. New York and London: Routledge

1991. *Simians, Cyborgs and Women: The reinvention of nature*. New York: Routledge

1992a. The Promises of Monsters: A regenerative politics for inappropriate/d others. In Lawrence Grossberg, Cary Nelson and Paula Treichler (eds.), *Cultural Studies*, pp. 295–337. New York: Routledge

1992b. When Man™ Is on the Menu. In Jonathon Crary and Sanford Kwinter (eds.), *Incorporations*, pp. 38–43. New York: Zone Books

1997. *Modest_Witness@Second_Millennium. FemaleMan©_Meets_OncoMouse™: Feminism and technoscience*. New York and London: Routledge

2003. *The Companion Species Manifesto: Dogs, people and significant otherness*. Chicago: Prickly Pear Press

Harding, Jennifer. 1997. Bodies at Risk: Sex, surveillance and hormone replacement therapy. In Alan Peterson and Robin Bunton (eds.), *Foucault, Health and Medicine*, pp. 134–50. London and New York: Routledge

Harding, Sandra, 1986. *The Science Question in Feminism*. Ithaca and London: Cornell University Press

1991. *Whose Science? Whose Knowledge? Thinking from women's lives*. Ithaca and New York: Cornell University Press

Harding, Sandra (ed.) 1993a. *The 'Racial' Economy of Science: Toward a democratic future*. Bloomington: Indiana University Press

Harding, Sandra. 1993b. Rethinking Standpoint Epistemology: What is 'strong objectivity'? In Linda Alcoff and Elizabeth Potter (eds.), *Feminist Epistomologies*, pp. 48–82. New York and London: Routledge

Hardon, Anita Petra. 1992. The Needs of Women Versus the Interests of Family Planning Personnel, Policy-makers and Researchers: Conflicting views on safety and acceptability of contraceptives. *Social Science and Medicine* 35(6): 735–66

Harris, Tess J., Cook, Derek, Wicks, Paul D. and Cappuccio, Francesco P. 1999. Ethnic Differences in Use of Hormone Replacement Therapy: Community based survey. *British Medical Journal* 319: 610–11

Hartouni, Valerie. 1997. *Cultural Conceptions: On reproductive technologies and the remaking of life*. Minneapolis and London: University of Minnesota Press

Hassler, Marianne. 1992. Creative Musical Behaviour and Sex Hormones: Musical talent and spatial ability in the two sexes. *Psychoneuroendocrinology* 17(1): 55–70

Hausman, Bernice. 1995. *Changing Sex: Transsexualism, technology and the idea of gender*. Durham, NC and London: Duke University Press

Hayles, N. Katherine. 1999. *How We Became Posthuman: Virtual bodies in cybernetics, literature and informatics*. Chicago: University of Chicago Press

Health Promotion England. 2000. *The Menopause: The facts about the menopause, HRT and osteoporosis*. London: Health Promotion England

Helén, Ilpo. 2004. Technics Over Life: Risk, ethics and the existential condition in high-tech antenatal care. *Economy and Society* 33(1): 28–51

Henwood, Flis, Wyatt, Sally, Hart, Angie and Smith, Julie. 2003. 'Ignorance is Bliss Sometimes': Constraints on the emergence of the 'informed patient' in the changing landscapes of health information. *Sociology of Health and Illness* 25(6): 589–607

Hersh, Adam L., Stefanick, Marcia L., Stafford, Randall S. 2004. National Use of Postmenopausal Hormone Therapy: Annual trends and response to recent evidence. *Journal of the American Medical Association* 291: 47–53

Hess, Rex A., Bunick, David and Bahr, Janice. 2001. Oestrogen, its Receptors and Function in the Male Reproductive Tract: A review. *Molecular and Cellular Endocrinology* 178(1–2): 29–38

Hill, Amelia. 2002. Damning Study on HRT Leaves Women in Limbo. *The Observer* 14 July. www.guardian.co.uk/medicine/story/0,,754950,00.html. Last accessed 25 September 2006

Hillard, T. 1997. Evaluation and Management of the Hormone Replacement (HRT) Candidate [review]. *International Journal of Fertility and Women's Medicine* 42 (Suppl. 2): 347–64

Hines, Melissa. 1998. Abnormal Sexual Development and Psychosexual Issues. *Ballière's Clinical Endocrinology and Metabolism* 12(1): 173–89

Hinshaw, Kim. 1996. May Depend on Whether the Menopause is Regarded as Physiological or Pathological [letter]. *British Medical Journal* 313: 686

Hird, Myra J. 2004. *Sex, Gender and Science*. Hampshire and New York: Palgrave Macmillan

Hirschbein, Laura. 2000. The Glandular Solution: Sex, masculinity and aging in the 1920s. *Journal of the History of Sexuality* 9(3): 277–304

Hirschfeld, Magnus. 1936. Homosexuality. In Victor Robinson (ed.), *Encyclopaedia Sexualis: A comprehensive encyclopaedia of the sexual sciences*, pp. 321–34. New York: Dingwall-Rock

Hoberman, John M. and Yesalis, Charles E. 1995. The History of Synthetic Testosterone. *Scientific American* February: 60–5

Hodann, Max. 1937. *History of Modern Morals*. Stella Browne (trans.). London: William Heineman (Medical Books)

Hoffman, Mikael, Lindh-Åstran, Lotta, Ahlner, Johan, Hammar, Mats and Kjellgren, Karin I. 2005. Hormone Replacement Therapy in the Menopause: Structure and content of risk talk. *Maturitas* 50(1): 8–15

Hogle, Linda. 2005. Enhancement Technologies and the Body. *Annual Review of Anthropology* 34: 695–716

Holmes, Morgan. 2000. Queer Cut Bodies. In Joseph A. Boone *et al.* (eds.), *Queer Frontiers: Millennial geographies, genders and generations*, pp. 84–110. Madison, WI and London: University of Wisconsin Press

hooks, bell. 1990. *Yearning: Race, gender and cultural politics*. Boston: South End Press.

Hope, Jenny. 2002. Taking Soy as HRT Substitute 'A Waste'. *Daily Mail Wednesday* 7 July. 39

Hunter, Myra S., O'Dea, Irene and Britten, Nicky. 1997. Decision-making and Hormone Replacement Therapy: A qualitative analysis. *Social Science and Medicine* 45(10): 1541–8

Irigaray, Luce. 1985. *This Sex Which Is Not One*. Catherine Porter and Carolyn Burke (trans.). Ithaca: Cornell University Press

  1993a. *Je, Tu, Nous: Toward a culture of sexual difference*. Alison Martin (trans.). New York and London: Routledge

  1993b. *An Ethics of Sexual Difference*. Carolyn Burke and Gillian C. Gill (trans.). Ithaca and New York: Cornell University Press

Irvine, Janice M. 1990. *Disorders of Desire: Sex and gender in modern American sexology*. Philadelphia: Temple University Press

Kaiser, Fran. E. 1991. Sexuality and Impotence in the Aging Man. *Clinics in Geriatric Medicine* 7(1): 63–75

Katz, Stephen and Marshall, Barbara. 2003. New Sex for Old: Lifestyle, consumerism, and the ethics of aging well. *Journal of Aging Studies* 17: 3–16

Kaufert, Patricia. 1982. Myth and the Menopause. *Sociology of Health and Illness* 4(2): 141–66

Kaufman, Jean Marc and Vermeulen, Alex. 1997. Declining Gonadal Function in Elderly Men. *Clinical Endocrinology and Metabolism* 11(20): 289–309

Kay, Lily. 2000. *Who Wrote the Book of Life? A history of the genetic code*. Stanford University Press

Keller, Evelyn Fox. 1995. *Reflections on Gender and Science* (Tenth Anniversary edn). New Haven and London: Yale University Press

  2001. *The Century of the Gene*. Cambridge, MA: Harvard University Press

Kenen, Stephanie H. 1997. Who Counts When You're Counting Homosexuals? Hormones and homosexuality in mid-twentieth century America. In Vernon A. Rosario (ed.), *Science and Homosexualities*, pp. 197–218. New York: Routledge

Kessler, Suzanne J. 1990. The Medical Construction of Gender: Case management of intersexed infants. *Signs: Journal of Women in Culture and Society* 16(1): 3–26

Kessler, Suzanne J. and McKenna, Wendy. 1978. *Gender: An ethnomethodological approach*. University of Chicago Press

Klein, Renate and Dumble, Lynette J. 1994. Disempowering Midlife Women: The science and politics of hormone replacement therapy (HRT). *Women's Studies International Forum* 17(4): 327–43

Konrad, Monica. 2005. *Narrating the New Genetics: Ethics, ethnography and science*. Cambridge University Press

Krieger, Nancy and Fee, Elizabeth. 1996. Man-made Medicine and Women's Health: The biopolitics of sex/gender and race/ethnicity. In Kary L. Moss (ed.), *Man-Made Medicine: Women's health, public policy and reform*, pp. 15–35. Durham, NC and London: Duke University Press

Krimsky, Sheldon. 2000. *Hormonal Chaos: The scientific and social origins of the environmental endocrine hypothesis.* Baltimore and London: The Johns Hopkins University Press

Kristeva, Julia. 1982. *Powers of Horror: An essay on abjection.* Leon S. Roudiez (trans.). New York: Columbia University Press

Kwok, Wei Leng. 1997. Menopause and the Great Divide: Biomedicine, feminism and cyborg politics. In Paul Komesaroff, Phillipa Rothfield and Jeanne Daly (eds.), *Reinterpreting Menopause: Cultural and philosophical issues,* pp. 255–72. New York and London: Routledge

LaCheen, Cary. 1986. Population Control and the Pharmaceutical Industry. In Kathleen McDonnell (ed.), *Adverse Effects: Women and the pharmaceutical industry,* pp. 89–136. Penang, Malaysia: International Organization of Consumers Unions Regional Office for Asia and the Pacific

Lam, P. M., Chung, T. K., and Haines, C. 2005. Where Are We With Postmenopausal Hormone Replacement Therapy in 2005? *Gynecological Endocrinology* 21(5): 248–56

Laqueur, Thomas. 1992. *Making Sex: Body and gender from the Greeks to Freud.* Cambridge, MA: Harvard University Press

Latour, Bruno. 1983. Give Me a Laboratory and I Will Raise the World. In Karin D. Knorr-Cetina and Michael Mulkay (eds.), *Science Observed: Perspectives on the social study of science,* pp. 141–70. London: Sage

1988. *The Pasteurization of France.* Alan Sheridan and John Law (trans.). Cambridge, MA: Harvard University Press

1990. Postmodern? No, simply amodern! Steps toward an anthropology of science. *Studies in the History and Philosophy of Science* 21(1): 145–51

1993. *We Have Never Been Modern.* Catherine Porter (trans.). Cambridge, MA: Harvard University Press

Latour, Bruno and Woolgar, Steve. 1979. *Laboratory Life: The social construction of scientific facts.* Beverley Hills and London: Sage

Laurance, Jeremy. 2003. HRT 'The New Thalidomide', Says Health Chief. *The Independent* 4 October: 1

Lauretis, Teresa de. 1994. The Essence of the Triangle or, Taking the Risk of Essentialism Seriously: Feminist theory in Italy, the U.S, and Britain. In Naomi Schor and Elizabeth Weed (eds.), *The Essential Difference,* pp. 1–39. Bloomington and Indianapolis: Indiana University Press

Lawrence, Felicity. 2004. Food Chained. *Chemical World Supplement, The Guardian* 15 May: 4–7

LeDoeuff, Michèle. 1989. *The Philosophical Imaginary.* Colin Gordon (trans.). London: The Athlone Press

Legros, J. J. 2000. Towards a Consensus Regarding Androgen Substitution Therapy for Andropause. *Review Medicine Liege* 55(5): 449–53

LeVay, Simon. 1991. Evidence for Anatomical Difference in the Brains of Homosexual Men. *Science* 253: 1034–7

1993. *The Sexual Brain.* Cambridge, MA: MIT Press

Leysen, Bettina. 1996. Medicalization of the Menopause: From 'Feminine Forever' to 'Healthy Forever'. In Nina Lykke and Rosi Braidotti (eds.), *Between*

Monsters, Goddesses and Cyborgs: Feminist confrontations with science, medicine and cyberspace, pp. 173–91. London: Zed Books

Lock, Margaret. 1993. *Encounters with Aging: Mythologies of menopause in Japan and North America*. Berkeley, LA and London: University of California Press

Lombardi, G., Zarrilli, S., Colao, A., Oaesano, L., Di Somma, C., Rossi, F. and De Rosa, M. 2001. Estrogens and Health in Males. *Molecular and Cellular Endocrinology* 178(1–2): 51–5

Longino, Helen and Doell, Ruth. 1983. Body, Bias and Behavior: A comparative analysis of reasoning in two areas of biological science. *Signs: A Journal of Women in Culture and Society* 9(2): 206–27

Luckas, Murray J. M, Gleeve, Toni, Biljan, Marinnko M., Buckett, William M., Aird, Ian A., Drakeley, Andrew and Kingland, Charles R. 1998. The Effects of Progestagens on the Carotid Artery Pulsatility Index in Postmenopausal Women on Oestrogen Replacement Therapy. *European Journal of Obstetrics and Gynecology and Reproductive Biology* 76: 221–4

Lund, B. C., Bever-Stille, K. A. and Perry, P. J. 1999. Testosterone and Andropause: The feasibility of testosterone replacement therapy in elderly men. *Pharmacotherapy* 19(8): 951–6

Lupton, Deborah. 1996. Constructing the Menopausal Body: The discourses on hormone replacement therapy. *Body and Society* 2(1): 91–7

Lykke, Nina. 1996. Between Monsters, Goddesses and Cyborgs: Feminist confrontations with science. In Nina Lykke and Rosi Braidotti (eds.), *Between Monsters, Goddesses and Cyborgs: Feminist confrontations with science, medicine and cyberspace*, pp. 13–29. London: Zed Books

Lynn, Richard. 1990. Testosterone and Gonadotropin Levels and r/K Reproductive Strategies. *Psychological Reports* 67: 1203–6

Lyons, Antonia C. and Griffin, Christine. 2003. Managing Menopause: A qualitative analysis of self-help literature for women at midlife. *Social Science and Medicine* 56: 1629–42

Maclennan, A. H., Taylor, A. W. and Watson, D. H. 1995. Changes in the Use of Hormone Replacement Therapy in South Australia. *Medical Journal of Australia* 162(8): 420–2

Mackenzie, Adrian. 2006. *Cutting Code: Software and sociality*. New York: Peter Lang

Madden, Richard. 1994. *Women's Health*. Canberra: Australian Bureau of Statistics

Maddley, Richard and Finnegan, Judy. 2002. HRT is a Change for the Better. *Daily Express* 11 May: 15

Mamo, L. and Fishman, J. 2001. Potency in All the Right Places: Viagra as a gendered technology of the body. *Body and Society* 7 (4): 13–35

Markowitz, Sally. 2001. Pelvic Politics: Sexual dimorphism and racial difference. *Signs: Journal of Women in Culture and Society* 26(2): 389–414

Marsh, Beezy. 2002. Why the HRT Generation Has a Fun-filled Life. *Daily Mail* 8 May: 30

Marshall, Barbara L. 2002. 'Hard Science': Gendered constructions of sexual dysfunction in the 'Viagra Age'. *Sexualities* 5: 131–58

Marshall, Barbara L. and Katz, Stephen. 2002. Forever Functional: Sexual fitness and the ageing male body. *Body and Society* 8(4): 43–70

Martin, Biddy. 1996. *Femininity Played Straight: The significance of being lesbian.* New York and London: Routledge

Martin, Emily. 1987. *The Woman in the Body: A cultural analysis of reproduction.* Boston: Beacon Press

1995. *Flexible Bodies: The role of immunity in American culture from the days of polio to the age of AIDS.* Boston: Beacon Press

1997. The Woman in the Menopausal Body. In Paul Komesaroff, Phillipa Rothfield and Jeanne Daly (eds.), *Reinterpreting Menopause: Cultural and philosophical issues*, pp. 239–54. New York and London: Routledge

2000a. The Rationality of Mania. In Roddey Reid and Sharon Traweek (eds.), *Doing Science + Culture*, pp. 177–98. New York and London: Routledge

2000b. Flexibility and Health. In Simon Willams, Jonathon Gave and Michal Calnan (eds.), *Health, Medicine and Society.* London and New York: Routledge

Mastrogiacomo I., Feghali, G., Foresta, C. and Ruzza, G. 1982. Andropause: Incidence and pathogenesis. *Archives of Andrology* 9: 293–6

McCormick, Cheryl M., Witelson, Sandra F. and Kingstone, Edward. 1990. Left-handedness in Homosexual Men and Women: Neuroendocrine implications. *Psychoneuroendocrinology* 15(1): 69–76

McCrea, Frances B. 1983. The Politics of Menopause: The 'discovery' of a deficiency disease. *Social Problems* 31(1): 109–23

McEwan, Bruce S. 2001. Genome and Hormones: Gender differences in physiology. Invited Review: Estrogens' effects on the brain: multiple sites and molecular mechanisms. *Journal of Applied Physiology* 91: 2785–801

McLachlan, John A. 2001. Environmental Signaling: What embryos and evolution teach us about endocrine disrupting chemicals. *Endocrine Reviews* 22(3): 319–41

McLaughlin, Dorothy. 2001. Silent Spring Revisited. www.pbs.org/wgbh/pages/frontline/shows/nature/disrupt/sspring.html. Last accessed 18 March 2007

M'charek, Amade. 2005. *The Human Genome Diversity Project: An ethnography of scientific practice.* Cambridge University Press

Medvei, Victor Cornelius. 1982. *A History of Endocrinology.* Lancaster, UK: MTP Press

Meikle, James. 2003. HRT Treatment Doubles Risk of Breast Cancer: Study of Million Women Sounds Warning. *The Guardian*, 8 August: 1

2005. Oestrogen Levels Need Pre-Menopause Boost to Thwart Heart Disease, Says Study. *The Guardian*, 9 December: 9

Millett, Kate. 1970. *Sexual Politics.* Garden City, NY: Doubleday and Co.

Mitteness, Linda S. 1983. Historical Changes in Public Information about the Menopause. *Urban Anthropology* 12(2): 161–72

Moir, Anne and Jessel, David. 1991. *Brain Sex: The real differences between men and women.* London: Mandarin

Mol, Annemarie. 2002. *The Body Multiple: Ontology in medical practice.* Durham, NC and London: Duke University Press

Mol, Annemarie and Law, John. 1994. Regions, Networks and Fluids: Anemia and social topology. *Social Studies of Science* 24: 641–71

Mol, Annemarie and Mesman, Jessica. 1996. Neonatal Food and the Politics of Theory: Some questions of method. *Social Studies of Science* 26: 419–44

Money, John. 1976. The Development of Sexology as a Discipline. *Journal of Sex Research* 12(2): 83–7

1982. Sexosophy: A new concept. *Journal of Sex Research* 18(4): 364–6

Moore, Celia L. 1984. Maternal Contributions to the Development of Masculine Sexual Behaviour in Laboratory Rats. *Developmental Psychobiology* 17: 347–56

Moore, Celia L. and Hui Dou. 1996. Number, Size, and Regional Distribution of Motor Neurons in the Dorsolateral and Retrodorsolateral Nuclei as a Function of Sex and Neonatal Stimulation. *Developmental Psychobiology* 29(4): 303–13

Moore, Celia L. and Power, Karen L. 1986. Prenatal Stress Eliminates Differential Maternal Attention to Male Offspring in Norway Rats. *Developmental Psychobiology* 38(5): 667–71

1992. Variation in Maternal Care and Individual Differences in Play, Exploration, and Grooming of Juvenile Norway Rat Offspring. *Developmental Psychobiology* 25(3): 165–82

Moore, Celia L., Wong, Lisa, Daum, Mary C. and Leclair, Ojingwa U. 1997. Mother–Infant Interactions in Two Strains of Rats: Implication for dissociating mechanism and function of a maternal pattern. *Developmental Psychobiology* 30(4): 310–2

Moorhead, Joanna. 2004. Pass on the Sweets. *Chemical World Supplement, The Guardian* 15 May: 20–3

Morales, Alvaro, Johnston, Brenda, Heaton, Jeremy P. and Lundie, Mark. 1997. Testosterone Supplementation for Hypogonadal Impotence: Assessment of biochemical measures and therapeutic outcomes. *Journal of Urology* 157 (March): 849–54

Morely, John E. 1991. Endocrine Factors in Geriatric Sexuality. *Clinics in Geriatric Medicine* 7(1): 85–93

2000. Andropause, Testosterone Therapy, and Quality of Life in Aging Men. *Cleveland Clinical Journal of Medicine* 67(12): 880–2

2001. Andropause: Is it time for the geriatrician to treat it? *Journals of Gerontology Series A: Biological Sciences and Medical Sciences* 56: 263–5

Morrison, Keith. 2004. The HRT Horses: What happens when the market dries up? Dateline NBC News, www.msnbc.msn.com/id/3995076/%20. Last accessed 25 September 2006

Moscucci, Ornella. 1990. *The Science of Woman: Gynaecology and gender in England, 1800–1929.* Cambridge University Press

Murray, Jenni. 2001. *Is it Me, or Is it Hot in Here? A modern woman's guide to the menopause.* London: Vermillion

Murtagh, Madeleine J. and Hepworth, Julie. 2003a Menopause as a Long-Term Risk to Health: Implications of general practitioner accounts of prevention for women's choice and decision-making. *Sociology of Health and Illness* 25(2): 185–207

2003b. Feminist Ethics and Menopause: Autonomy and decision-making in primary medical care. *Social Science and Medicine* 5: 1643–52

Myers, Greg. 1990. *Writing Biology: Texts in the social construction of scientific knowledge.* Madison, WI: University of Wisconsin Press

National Institutes of Health. 2002. NHLBI Stops Trial of Estrogen Plus Progestin due to Increased Breast Cancer Risk, Lack of Overall Benefit. NIH News Release, 9 July, www.nhlbi.nih.gov/new/press/02-07-09.htm. Last accessed 25 September 2006

National Research Council. 1999. *Hormonally Active Agents in the Environment.* Washington, DC: National Academy Press

Neave, Nick and Menaged, Meyrav. 1999. Sex Differences in Cognition: The role of testosterone and sexual orientation. *Brain and Cognition* 41: 245–62

Neischlag, E. 1996. Testosterone Replacement Therapy: Something old, something new. *Clinical Endocrinology* 45(3): 261–2

Nelkin, Dorothy. 1987. *Selling Science: How the press covers science and technology.* New York: W. H. Freeman and Company

Newbold, R. R., Hanson, R. B., Jefferson, W. N., Bullock, B. C., Haseman, J. and McLachlan, J. A. 1998. Increased Tumors but Uncompromised Fertility in the Female Descendants of Mice Exposed Developmentally to Diethylstilbestrol. *Carcinogenesis* 19(9): 1655–63

Novas, Carlos and Rose, Nikolas. 2000. Genetic Risk and the Birth of the Somatic Individual. *Economy and Society* 29(4): 485–513

Novo Nordisk n.d. Choosing HRT: Weighing up the facts. KV/01/72

—— 1993. Trisquens® advertisement. *Modern Medicine: The Journal of Clinical Medicine* 36(3)

Nye, Robert A. 2005. Locating Masculinity: Some recent work on men. *Signs: A Journal of Women in Culture and Society* 30(3) Spring: 1937–62

Oakley, Ann. 1972. *Sex, Gender and Society,* London: Temple Smith

O'Connor, Ahmad. 2004. Sex on the Brain – It Depends on the Gender. *Sydney Morning Herald* 25 March: 7

Oddens, B. J., Boulet, P., Lehert P. and Visser, P. 1992. Has the Climacteric Been Medicalized? A study on the use of medication for climacteric complaints in four countries. *Maturitas* 15(3): 171–81

Oudshoorn, Nelly. 1994. *Beyond the Natural Body: An archeology of sex hormones.* New York and London: Routledge

—— 1996a. A Natural Order of Things? Reproductive sciences and the politics of othering. In George Robertson, Melinda Mash, Lisa Tickner, Jon Bird, Barry Curtis and Tim Putnam (eds.), *FutureNatural: Nature, science, culture,* pp. 122–32. London and New York: Routledge

—— 1996b. The Decline of the One-Size-Fits-All Paradigm, or How Reproductive Scientists Try to Cope with Postmodernity. In Nina Lykke and Rosi Braidotti (eds.), *Between Monsters, Goddesses and Cyborgs: Feminist confrontations with science, medicine and cyberspace,* pp. 153–72. London: Zed Books

—— 2003. *The Male Pill: A biography of a technology in the making.* Durham, NC and London: Duke University Press

Palmert, M. R. and Boepple, P. A. 2001. Variation in the Timing of Puberty: Clinical spectrum and genetic investigation. *Journal of Clinical Endocrinology and Metabolism* 86(6): 2364–8

Palmund, I. 1997. The Marketing of Estrogens for Menopausal and Postmenopausal Women. *Journal of Psychosomatic Obstetrics and Gynaecology* 19: 158–64

Polo-Kantola, P., Portin, R., Polo, O., Helenius, H., Irjala, K. and Erkkola, R. 1998. The Effect of Short-term Estrogen Replacement Therapy on Cognition: A randomized, double-blind, crossover trial in postmenopausal women. *Obstetrics and Gynecology* 91(3): 459–66

Porter, Roy and Hall, Lesley. 1995. *The Facts of Life: The creation of sexual knowledge in Britain, 1650–1950*. New Haven and London: Yale University Press

Potts, Annie. 2004. Deleuze on Viagra (Or, What Can a Viagra-body Do?). *Body and Society* 10(1): 17–36

Potts, Annie, Gavey, Nicola, Grace, Victoria M. and Vares, Tiina. 2003. The Downsides of Viagra: Women's experiences and concerns. *Sociology of Health and Illness* 25(7): 697–719

Prevelic, Gordana and Jacobs, Howard S. 1997. Menopause and Postmenopause. *Clinical Endocrinology and Metabolism* 11(2): 313–40

Prior, Jerilynn C., Vigna, Yvette M. and Watson, Diane. 1989. Spironolactone with Physiological Female Steroids for Presurgical Therapy of Male-to-Female Transsexualism. *Archives of Sexual Behaviour* 18(1): 49–57

Rabinow, Paul. 1992. Artificiality and Enlightenment: From sociobiology to biosociality. In J. Crary and S. Kwinter (eds.), *Incorporations*, pp. 234–52. New York: Zone Books

1999. *French DNA: Trouble in purgatory*. University of Chicago Press.

Raloff, Janet. 1994a. The Gender Benders: Are environmental 'hormones' emasculating wildlife? *Science News* 145(2) 8 Jan.: 24–7

1994b. That Feminine Touch: Are men suffering from prenatal or childhood exposures to 'hormonal toxicants?' *Science News* 145(4) 22 Jan: 56–8

Rapp, Rayna. 1999. *Testing Women, Testing the Fetus*. New York and London: Routledge

Rapp, Rayna and Ginsburg, Faye. 2001. Enabling Disability: Rewriting kinship, reimagining citizenship. *Public Culture* 13(3): 533–56

Rapp, Rayna, Heath, Deborah and Taussig, Karen-Sue. 2001. Genealogical Disease: Where hereditary abnormality, biomedical explanation, and family responsibility meet. In Sarah Franklin and Susan McKinnon (eds.), *Relative Values: Reconfiguring kinship studies*, pp. 384–412. Durham, NC: Duke University Press

Rayner, Claire. 2002. Why it Is Worth Taking the Risk. *The Guardian*, 11 July, www.guardian.co.uk/medicine/story/0,,753117,00.html. Last accessed 26 September 2006

Reeve, J. 1992. Future Prospects for Hormone Replacement Therapy. *British Medical Bulletin* 48(2): 458–68

Reinisch, June Macover, Ziemba-Davis, Mary and Sanders, Stephanie A. 1991. Hormonal Contributions to Sexually Dimorphic Behavioral Development in Humans. *Psychoneuroendocrinology* 16 (1–3): 213–78

Reuben, David. 1971. *Everything You Always Wanted to Know About Sex But Were Afraid to Ask*. London: Pan Books

Riley, Denise. 1988. *Am I That Name? Feminism and the category of 'women' in history*. Minneapolis: University of Minnesota Press

Riley, Pete, Bell, Sandra and Warhurst, Michael. 1999. Briefing: Endocrine disrupting chemicals. Friends of the Earth, www.foe.co.uk/resource/briefings/endocrine_disrupting.html. Last accessed 25 September 2006

Roberts, Celia. 2000. Biological Behavior? Hormones, psychology and sex. *The Science and Politics of the Search for Sex Differences: A special issue of the NWSA journal* 12(3): 1–20

2002a. 'Successful Aging' with Hormone Replacement Therapy: It may be sexist, but what if it works? *Science as Culture* 11(1): 39–59

2002b. 'A Matter of Embodied Fact': Sex hormones and the history of bodies. *Feminist Theory* 3(1): 7–26

2003a. Sex, Race and 'Unnatural' Difference: Tracking the chiastic logic of meno-pause-related discourses. *European Journal of Women's Studies* 11(1): 27–44

2003b. Drowning in a Sea of Estrogens: Sex hormones, sexual reproduction and sex. *Sexualities* 6(2): 195–213

Roberts, Celia and Franklin, Sarah. 2005. Experiencing New Forms of Genetic Choice: Findings from an ethnographic study of preimplantation genetic diagnosis. *Human Fertility* 7(4): 285–294

Roberts, Celia and Mackenzie, Adrian. 2006. Science: Experimental sensibilities in practice. *Theory, Culture and Society* 23(2–3): 137–62

Rochira, Vincenzo, Balestrieri, Antonio, Madeo, Bruno, Baraldi, Enrica, Faustini-Fustini, Marco, Granata, Antonio R. M. and Carani, Cesare. 2001. Congenital Estrogen Deficiency: In search of the Estrogen role in human male reproduction. *Molecular and Cellular Endocrinology* 178(1–2): 107–15

Rogers, Lesley J. 1988. Biology, the Popular Weapon: Sex differences in cognitive function. In Barbara Caine, E. A. Grosz and Marie deLepervanche (eds.), *Crossing Boundaries: Feminisms and the critique of knowledges*, pp. 43–51. Sydney: Allen and Unwin

1998. Indirect Influences of Gonadal Hormones on Sexual Differentiation. *Behavioral and Brain Sciences* 21(3): 337–8

1999. *Sexing the Brain.* London: Weidenfield and Nicolson

Rose, Nikolas. 2001. The Politics of Life Itself. *Theory, Culture and Society* 18(6): 1–30

Royal Society, the. 2000. *Endocrine disrupting chemicals (EDCs).* June. London: The Royal Society

Rubin, Gayle. 1994. Sexual Traffic: Interview with Judith Butler. *Differences: A Journal of Feminist Cultural Studies* 6(2–3): 62–99

Russell, Andrew and Thompson, Mary S. 2000. Introduction: Contraception across cultures. In Andrew Russell, Elisa J. Sobo and Mary S. Thompson (eds.), *Contraception Across Cultures: Technologies, choices, constraints*, pp. 3–25. Oxford and New York: Berg

Russell, Andrew, Sobo, Elisa J. and Thompson, Mary S. (eds.) 2000. *Contraception Across Cultures: Technologies, choices, constraints.* Oxford and New York: Berg

Russett, Cynthia Eagle. 1989. *Sexual Science: The Victorian construction of woman-hood.* Cambridge, MA: Harvard University Press

Sample, Ian. 2006. Free IVF for All Would Ease Pensions Crisis, Say Researchers. *The Guardian* 20 June: 11

Schiebinger, Londa. 1989. *The Mind Has No Sex? Women in the origins of modern science.* Cambridge, MA: Harvard University Press

1993. *Nature's Body: Sexual politics and the making of modern science.* London: Pandora

Seaman, Barbara. 2003. *The Greatest Experiment Ever Performed on Women: Exploding the oestrogen myth.* New York: Hyperion

Seaman, Barbara and Seaman, Gideon. 1977. *Women and the Crisis in Sex Hormones.* New York: Bantam

Sedgwick, Eve Kososky. 1991. *Epistemology of the Closet.* Berkeley, CA: University of California Press

Sengoopta, Chandak. 1998. Glandular Politics: Experimental biology, clinical medicine, and homosexual emancipation in *fin-de-siècle* Central Europe. *Isis* 89: 445–473

2000. The Modern Ovary: Constructions, meanings, uses. *History of Science* 38(4), no. 122: 425–88

Serres, Michel, with Latour, Bruno. 1995. *Conversations on Science, Culture and Time.* Roxanne Lapidus (trans.) Ann Arbor: University of Michigan Press

Shapin, Steven and Shaffer, Simon. 1985. *Leviathan and the Air-pump: Hobbes, Boyle, and the experimental life.* Princeton University Press

Sharpe, Richard M. and Irvine, D. Stewart. 2004. How Strong Is the Evidence of a Link Between Environmental Chemicals and Adverse Effects on Human Reproductive Health? *British Medical Journal* (328) (21 February): 447–51

Shaw, J. M. and Snow, C. M. 1998. Weighted Vest Exercise Improves Indices of Fall Risk in Older Women. *Journal of Gerontology Series A: Biological and Medical Sciences* 53(1): 53–8

Sherwin, Barbara. 1998. Estrogen and Cognitive Functioning in Women. *Proceedings of the Society for Experimental Biology and Medicine* 217(1): 17–22

Sherwood, Lauralee. 1989. *Human Physiology: From cells to systems.* St. Paul, MI: West Publishing Company

1997. *Human Physiology: From cells to systems.* 2nd edition. St. Paul, MI: West Publishing Company

2007. *Human Physiology: From cells to systems,* 6th edn. Belmont, CA: Thomson, Brooks/Cole

Shippen and Fryer, 1998. *The Testostone Syndrome: The critical factor for energy, health, and sexuality – reversing the male menopause.* New York: M. Evans and Company

Shorett, Peter. 2002. Of Transgenic Mice and Men. *GeneWatch* 15(5) September. www.gene-watch.org/genewatch/articles/15-5mice.html. Last accessed 25 September 2006

Singleton, Vicky. 1996. Feminism, Sociology of Scientific Knowledge and Postmodernism: Politics, theory and me. *Social Studies of Science* 26: 445–68

Slabbekoorn, Ditte, van Goozen, Stephanie H. M., Sanders, Geofff, Gooren, Louis J. G. and Cohen-Kettenis, Peggy T. 2000. The Dermatoglyphic Characteristics of Transsexuals: Is there evidence for an organizing effect of sex hormones. *Psychoneuroendocrinology* 25: 365–75

Smith-Rosenberg, Carroll. 1989. Discourses of Sexuality and Subjectivity: The new woman, 1870–1936. In Martin Bauml Duberman, Martha Vicinus and George Chauncy, Jr. (eds), *Hidden from History: Reclaiming the gay and lesbian past,* pp. 264–80. New York: NAL Books

Solomon, Gina M. and Schettler, Ted. 2000. Environment and Health: 6. Endocrine disruption and potential human health implications. *Canadian Medical Association Journal* 28 November, 163(11): 1471–6

Solstad, K. and Garde, K. 1992. Middle-aged Danish Men's Ideas of a Male Climacteric – and of the Female Climacteric. *Maturitas* 15(1): 7–16

Spanier, Bonnie B. 1995. *Im/partial Science: Gender ideology in molecular biology.* Bloomington and Indianapolis: Indiana University Press

Speroff, Leon. 1993. Menopause and Hormone Replacement Therapy. *Clinics in Geriatric Medicine* 9(1): 33–55

1997. Postmenopausal Hormone Therapy into the 21st Century. *International Journal of Gynecology and Obstetrics*, Suppl. 1: 3–10

Spivak, Gayatri Chakravorty, with Grosz, Elizabeth. 1984. Criticism, Feminism and the Institution. In Sarah Harasym (ed.), *The Post Colonial Critic: Interviews, strategies, dialogues / Gayatri Chakravorty Spivak*, pp. 1–16. New York: Routledge

Spivak, Gayatri Chakravorty, with Rooney, Ellen. 1994. In a Word. Interview. In Naomi Shor and Elizabeth Weed (eds.), *The Essential Difference*, pp. 151–84. Bloomington and Indianapolis: Indiana University Press

Stacey, Jackie. 1997. *Teratologies: A cultural study of cancer.* London and New York: Routledge

2000. The Global Within: Consuming nature, embodying health. In Sarah Franklin, Celia Lury, and Jackie Stacey, *Global Nature, Global Culture*, pp. 97–145. London: Sage Publications

Stanford, Janet L., Weiss, Noel S., Voigt, Lynda, Dalling, Janet R., Habel, Laurel A. and Rossing, Mary Anne. 1995. Combined Estrogen and Progestin Hormone Replacement Therapy in Relation to Risk of Breast Cancer in Middle-Aged Women. *Journal of the American Medical Association* 274(2): 137–42

Star, Susan Leigh. 1991. Power, Technology and the Phenomenology of Conventions: On being allergic to onions. In John Law (ed.), *A Sociology of Monsters? Power, technology and the modern world*, pp. 26–56. Sociological Review Monograph 38. Oxford: Basil Blackwell

Steakley, James D. 1997. *Per Scientiam Ad Justitiam*: Magnus Hirschfeld and the sexual politics of innate homosexuality. In Vernon Rosario (ed.), *Science and Homosexualities*, pp. 133–54. New York: Routledge

Steinach, Eugen and Loebel, Josef. 1940. *Sex and Life: Forty years of biological and medical experiments.* London: Faber and Faber

Stepan, Nancy. 1993. Race and Gender: The role of analogy in science. In Sandra Harding (ed.), *The 'Racial' Economy of Science: Toward a democratic future*, pp. 359–76. Bloomington and Indianapolis: Indiana University Press

Stepan, Nancy and Gilman, Sander. 1993. Appropriating the Idioms of Science: The rejection of scientific racism. In Sandra Harding (ed.), *The 'Racial' Economy of Science: Toward a democratic future*, pp. 170–93. Bloomington and Indianapolis: Indiana University Press

Stewart, Jane. 1988. Current Themes, Theoretical Issues, and Preoccupations in the Study of Sexual Differentiation and Gender-Related Behaviors. *Psychobiology* 16 (4): 315–20

Stone, Richard. 1994. Environmental Estrogens Stir Debate. *Science* 265: 308–10

Subbiah, M. T. 1998. Mechanisms of Cardioprotection by Estrogens. *Proceedings of the Society for Experimental Biology and Medicine* 217(1): 23–9

Suchman, Lucy. 1999. Working Relations of Technology Production and Use. In D. Mackenzie and J. Wajcman (eds.), *The Social Shaping of Technology*, 2nd edn, pp. 258–65. Buckingham, UK: Open University Press

Sultan, Charles, Balaguer, Terouanne, Béatrice, Georget, Virginie, Paris, François, Jeandel, Claire, Lumbroso, Serge and Nicolas, Jean-Claude. 2001. Environmental Xenoestrogens, Antiandrogens and Disorders of Male Sexual Differentiation. *Molecular and Cellular Endocrinology* 178(1–2): 99–105

Swaab, D. F. 2004. Sexual Differentiation of the Human Brain: Relevance for gender identity, transsexualism and sexual orientation. *Gynecology and Endocrinology* 19: 301–12

Sybylla, Roe. 1997. Situating Menopause within the Strategies of Power. In Paul Komesaroff, Phillipa Rothfield and Jeanne Daly (eds.), *Reinterpreting Menopause: Cultural and philosophical issues*, pp. 200–21. New York and London: Routledge

Takaki, Ronald T. 1993. Aesculapius Was a White Man: Race and the cult of true womanhood. In Sandra Harding (ed.), *The 'Racial' Economy of Science: Toward a democratic future*, pp. 201–9. Bloomington and Indianapolis: Indiana University Press

Tan, R. S. and Philip, P. S. 1999. Perceptions of and Risk Factors for Andropause. *Archives of Andrology* 43(3): 227–33

Teilman, Grete, Juul, Anders, Skakkebæk and Toppari, Jorma. 2002. Putative Effects of Endocrine Disrupters on Pubertal Development in the Human. *Best Practice and Research in Clinical Endocrinology and Metabolism* 16(1): 105–21

Terry, Jennifer. 1997. The Seductive Power of Science in the Making of Deviant Subjectivity. In Vernon A. Rosario (ed.), pp. 271–95. *Science and Homosexualities*. New York: Routledge

  1999. *An American Obsession: Science, medicine and homosexuality in modern society*. Chicago University Press

Thornton, Joe. 1997. *The PVC Lifecycle: Dioxin from cradle to grave*. Greenpeace U.S.A, April. http://archive.greenpeace.org/toxics/reports/reports.html

Throsby, Karen. 2004. *When IVF Fails: Feminism, infertility and the negotiation of normality*. Houndsmills and New York: Palgrave Macmillan

Tiefer, Leonore. 1994. Three Crises Facing Sexology. *Archives of Sexual Behavior* 23(4): 361–74

Topo, P., Koster, A., Holte, A., Collins, A., Landgren, B. M., Hemminki, E. and Uutela, A. 1995. Trends in the Use of Climacteric and Postclimacteric Hormones in Nordic Countries. *Maturitas* 22: 89–95

UC Davis Cancer Center. 2003. Of Mice and Women. *Synthesis: A publication of the UC Davis Cancer Center*, www.ucdmc.ucdavis.edu/synthesis/Archives/fall03/feature/feature.html. Last accessed 25 September 2006

Urry, John. 2003. *Global Complexity*. London: Polity

Utian, W. H. and Schiff, I. 1994. NAMS-Gallup Survey on Women's Knowledge, Information Sources, and Attitudes to Menopause and Hormone

Replacement Therapy. *Menopause: The Journal of the North American Menopause Society* 1(1): 39–48

Van de Graaf, Kent M. and Fox, Stuart Ira. 1989. *Concepts of Human Anatomy and Physiology.* 2nd edn. Dubuque, IA: Wm. C. Brown Publishers

Van den Wijngaard, Marianne. 1997. *Reinventing the Sexes: The biomedical construction of femininity and masculinity.* Bloomington and Indianapolis: Indiana University Press

Van Wingerden, Ineke. 1996. Postmodern Visions of the Menopausal Body: The apparatus of bodily production and the case of brittle bones. In Nina Lykke and Rosi Braidotti (eds.), *Between Monsters, Goddesses and Cyborgs: Feminist confrontations with science, medicine and cyberspace,* pp. 192–206. London: Zed Books

Vermeulen, A. 1993. The Male Climaterium. *Annuals of Medicine* 25(6): 531–44

2000. Andropause. *Maturitas* 34(1): 5–15

Verrell, Paul. 1991. Why Small Is Sometimes Sexy. *New Scientist* 7 September: 44–7

Vines, Gail. 1993. *Raging Hormones: Do they rule our lives?* London: Virago Press

Vreughenhil, Hestien J. I., Silpjer, Froukje M. E., Mulder, Paul G. H. and Weisglas-Kuperus, Nynke. 2002. Effects of Perinatal Exposure to PCBs and Dioxins on Play Behaviour in Dutch Children at School Age. *Environmental Health Perspectives* 110(10): 593–8

Waldby, Catherine. 1996. *AIDS and the Body Politic: Biomedicine and sexual difference.* London: Routledge

2000. *The Visible Human Project: Informatic bodies and posthuman medicine.* London: Routledge

2002. Stem Cells, Tissue Cultures and the Production of Biovalue. *Health* 6(3): 305–23

Warhurst, A. M. 2000. *Crisis in Chemicals.* London: Friends of the Earth.

Watson Pharma Inc. 1996. Androderm™ advertisement. *Endocrinology* 137(2)

Weed, Elizabeth. 1994. The Question of Style. In Carolyn Burke, Naomi Schor and Margaret Whitford (eds.), *Engaging with Irigaray: Feminist philosophy and modern European thought,* pp. 79–109. New York: Colombia University Press

Weeks, Jeffrey. 1981. *Sex, Politics and Society: The Regulation of sexuality since 1800.* London: Longman Group

1986. *Sexuality.* Chichester: Ellis Horwood

West M. J., White, D. J. and King, A. P. 2003. Female Brown-headed Cowbirds (Molothrus ater): Organization and behavior reflects male social dynamics. *Animal Behavior* 64: 377–85

Whitehead, Stephen M. and Barrett, Frank J. (eds.) 2001. *The Masculinities Reader.* Cambridge and Malden: Polity

Wiegman, Robyn. 1995. *American Anatomies: Theorizing race and gender.* Durham, NC: Duke University Press

Wilbush, Joel. 1979. La Menopausie: The birth of a syndrome. *British Medical Journal* 281(6239): 563–4

1981a. Climacteric Symptom Formation: Donovan's contribution. *Maturitas* 3(2): 99–105

1981b. What's in a Name? Some linguistic aspects of the climacteric. *Maturitas* 3(1): 1–9

1982. Historical perspectives: Climacteric expression and social context. *Maturitas* 4(3): 195–205

1985. Surveys of Climacteric Semiology in Non-western Populations: A critique. *Maturitas* 7(4): 289–96

1988a. Menopause and Menorrhagia: A historical exploration. *Maturitas* 10(2): 83–108

1988b. Menorrhagia and Menopause: A historical review. *Maturitas* 10(1): 5–26

1993. The Climacteric Kaleidoscope: Questions and speculations. *Maturitas* 16(3): 157–62

1994. Confrontation in the Climacteric. *Journal of the Royal Society of Medicine* 87(June): 342–7

Williams, Simon J. and Gillian Bendelow. 1998. *The Lived Body: Sociological themes, embodied issues*. New York and London: Routledge

Wilson, Elizabeth A. 1998. *Neural Geographies: Feminism and the microstructure of cognition*. New York: Routledge

1999. Introduction: Somatic Compliance – Feminism, Biology and Science. *Australian Feminist Studies* 14(29): 7–18

2004. *Psychosomatic: Feminism and the neurological body*. Durham, NC and London: Duke University Press

Wilson, Robert A. 1966. *Feminine Forever*. London: Mayflower Books

Winner, Langdon. 1993. Upon Opening the Black Box and Finding it Empty: Social constructivism and the philosophy of technology. *Science, Technology and Human Values* 18(3): 362–78

Witelson, Sandra F. 1991. Neural Sexual Mosaicism: Sexual differentiation of the human temporo-parietal region for functional asymmetry. *Psycho-neuroendocrinology* 16(1–3): 131–53

Wolff, Charlotte. 1986. *Magnus Hirshfeld: A portrait of a pioneer in sexology*. London: Quartet Books

Wolpert, Lewis. 1993. *The Triumph of the Embryo*. Oxford University Press

Woodward, Katherine. 1991. *Aging and its Discontents: Freud and other fictions*. Bloomington and Indianapolis: Indiana University Press

1994. From Virtual Cyborgs to Biological Time Bombs: Technocriticism and the material body. In Gretchen Bender and Timothy Druckery (eds.), *Culture on the Brink: Ideologies of technology*, pp. 47–64. Seattle: Bay Press

Woolgar, Steve. 1993. Configuring the User: The case of usability trials. In John Law (ed.), *A Sociology of Monsters: Essays on Power, Technology and Domination*, pp. 57–98. London: Routledge

Worchester, Nancy and Whatley, Marianne M. 1992. The Selling of HRT: Playing on the fear factor. *Feminist Review* 41: 1–26

World Wild life Fund. 1998. Chemicals that Compromise Life: A call to action. www.worldwildlife.org/news/pubs/toxics/ctcl.htm. Last accessed 1 September 2004

1999. *Persistent Organic Pollutants: Hand-me-down poisons that threaten wildlife and people. Issue Brief*. Washington, DC http://worldwildlife.org/toxics/pubs/pop.pdf. Last accessed 25 September 2006

2000. *Reducing Your Risk: A UK guide to avoiding hormone disruptors*, Surrey: WWF. www.wwf.org.uk/filelibrary/pdf/risk.pdf. Last accessed 26 September 2006

2002. Who Cares Where Toxic Chemicals End Up? campaign. *Country Living* February: 43; *Observer Food Monthly* February 25; www.wwf.org.uk/ chemicals/about.asp. Last accessed 25 September 2006

2006. 'Toxic Chemicals'. http://worldwildlife.org/toxics/. Last accessed 2 October 2006

Writing Group for the Women's Health Initiative Randomized Controlled Trial. 2002. Risks and Benefits of Estrogen Plus Progestin in Healthy Post-menopausal Women. *Journal of the American Medical Association* 288(3): 321–3

Yaffe, K., Sawaya, G., Lieberburg, I. and Grady, D. 1998. Estrogen Therapy in Postmenopausal Women: Effects on function and dementia. *Journal of the American Medical Association* 279(9): 688–95

Young, Iris Marion. 1990. *Throwing Like a Girl and Other Essays in Feminist Philosophy*. Bloomington, IN: Indiana University Press

Zavos, P. M., Kaskar, K., Correa, J. R. and Sikka, S. C. 2006. Seminal Characteristics and Sexual Behavior in Men of Different Age Groups: Is there an aging effect? *Asian Journal of Andrology* 8(3): 337–41

Zumoff, Barnett. 1998. Does Postmenopausal Estrogen Administration Increase the Risk of Breast Cancer? Contributions of nimal, biochemical, and clinical investigative studies to a resolution of the controversy. *Proceedings of the Society for Experimental Biology and Medicine* 217(1): 30–7

Index

Printed in the United States
By Bookmasters